Your Best Health Under the Sun

Learn to Use the Natural Power of Sunlight and...

- **Cure Depression**
- **Beat Cancer**
- **Prevent Heart Disease**
- **Build Stronger Bones** ·
- **Live a Longer, Healthier Life**

Al Sears, M.D. & Jon Herring

With a Preface by Michael Masterson

Published by:
Al Sears, MD • 12794 Forest Hill Blvd., Suite 16 • Wellington, FL 33414
www.AlSearsMD.com

TABLE OF CONTENTS

How we benefited from our native sun for eons… why we recently began hiding from the sun… how sun avoidance takes its toll
mentally and physically… the crucial nutrient we need from sunlight… how to undo the biggest health mistake of the century.

Who demonized sunlight… who profits from fear of the sun…
how the Sun Police silence health professionals who advocate sun
exposure… the flawed studies used to create fear… how to cut
through the paranoia and safely take advantage of healthy sunlight.

How deficiency of the sunshine vitamin hurts your tissues and
organs… how your body uses sunlight to make your most powerful hormone… why you're most likely deficient… why your
body craves more sunlight… take this first step to recover from
deficiency.

Why vitamin D deficiency has become so widespread… how to
see its affects on you… how to safely get enough vitamin D from
the sun… what to do when the sunlight is not enough… why
synthetic vitamin D is a bad idea and how you can get the right
kind.

MEET THE AUTHORS

Dr. Al Sears

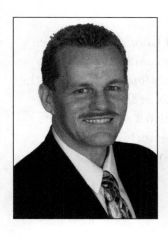

Al Sears, MD continues to see patients at his integrative clinic and research center in Florida where he has developed novel exercise and nutritional systems transforming the lives of over 20,000 patients.

His original contributions and commanding knowledge of alternative medicine have put him at the forefront of anti-aging medicine, both as a lecturer and published author.

His latest release, *PACE: Rediscover Your Native Fitness* sparked a revolution in the fitness world. An effective alternative to traditional cardio, PACE is practiced in 23 countries, delivering reliable fat loss and prevention against heart attack and stroke.

He has written over 500 articles and 6 books in the fields of alternative medicine, anti-aging and nutritional supplementation. He enjoys a worldwide readership and has appeared on over 50 national radio programs, ABC News, CNN and ESPN.

His third book, *The Doctor's Heart Cure*, exposed the real causes of the modern epidemic of heart disease with practical how-to advice for building real heart strength and resistance to disease without drugs. It is available in 9 languages and remains a best-seller 3 years after its publication.

In 2005, Dr. Sears' *12 Secrets to Virility* shed light on the huge environmental and nutritional problems with virility in our modern world, gave men a step-by step guide for maintaining health, strength and masculinity as they age, and became a bestseller during its first month of release.

He publishes a monthly newsletter – *Health Confidential* – addressing the issues of aging, nutrition and sexual health for men and women, a weekly e-letter called *Doctor's House Call* and is the health columnist to a circulation of hundreds of thousands in the popular self-help letter *Early to Rise*. He is also a member of the Health Sciences Institute Medical Advisory Panel.

Jon Herring

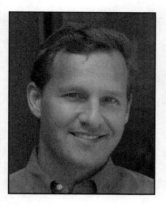

More than five years ago, Jon Herring began to realize that most of what we have been told about health, disease, food and medicine is just plain wrong. Since then Jon has invested thousands of hours to the study of health, fitness and nutrition. As the Health Editor of *Early to Rise*, Jon has written hundreds of articles to help others make more informed decisions about their own health.

In the course of his study, Jon began to learn just how vital the healing power of sunlight is to our bodies. It became clear that millions of people worldwide are suffering from poor health and disease, partly because we have become disconnected from our native sun. Jon has made it his mission to educate people about the vast number of health benefits that sunlight and vitamin D can provide.

In his research for the book, *Your Best Health Under the Sun*, a collaborative effort with Dr. Al Sears, Jon has reviewed more than 300 peer-reviewed studies, hundreds of articles and more than 10 books on the subject of vitamin D, light and health. It is his passion to share this life-saving information with as many people as possible and it was in this spirit that *Your Best Health Under the Sun* was written.

PREFACE

Americans like to think that we are among the healthiest people in the world. The truth is otherwise. If you subtract infant mortality and AIDS from the calculations, the average longevity of an Upper Voltan is only one year less than that of an American. That difference – that twelve-month difference – is the twelve months you spend in agony, pumped up with drugs and suffering from modern life extension medicine. That miserable additional lifespan consumes a ridiculously large percentage of what you spend on health.

Americans are unhealthy for a variety of reasons, but three of the most important ones are what we eat, how we exercise and how we relate to the sun.

Americans eat way too much artificial food that fails to provide nourishment, depletes our immune systems, and makes us fat. We also spend an amazing amount of time (6 hours a day on average!) sitting on our asses and watching television. That is bad. Really bad. And when we try to compensate for it by lifting weights and jogging, we do little more than damage our joints and reduce our muscularity.

We eat wrong and exercise badly because we have been given bad advice. But the worst advice we may have ever received is about the sun. For about 30 years now, Americans have been deluged with advertisements and deceived by the media about the role of sunlight and health.

Despite what our grandmothers told us, and notwithstanding a preponderance of scientific evidence, we have come to believe that the sun is our enemy. The truth is that the sun is the best friend we have when it comes to feeling good, staying fit and avoiding disease (including skin cancer). The sun is the answer!

In the pages that follow, Jon Herring and Dr. Al Sears explain why the sun may be the single most powerful disease fighter in the universe. The sun is our main source of vitamin D, an absolutely vital substance that:

- Helps to prevent 17 different deadly internal cancers
- Helps to prevent the deadly skin cancer melanoma
- Lowers the risk Type-1 and Type-2 diabetes
- Prevents autoimmune disorders like multiple sclerosis and rheumatoid arthritis
- Reduces the risk of heart attack
- Lowers cholesterol, blood pressure, and inflammation
- Boosts immunity and protects against cold and flu
- Increases the strength of your bones and prevents osteoporosis
- Reduces falls in the elderly
- Helps to prevent fibromyalgia
- Improves muscle function and reaction time
- Prevents depression and regulates mood
- Prevents cavities and tooth loss
- Prevents unexplained bone and muscle pain (including back pain)
- Increases fertility and boosts sex hormones in men and women
- Prevents inflammatory bowel disease and other digestive disorders

That's just a partial list. The complete list of benefits from vitamin D would take pages. And in every one of the conditions above you can substitute "helps to treat" in place of "helps to prevent." There is no question that if you are deficient in vitamin D, that you run the risk of meeting an early grave. And if you are already suffering poor health, a deficiency of vitamin D could be the reason.

Let me ask you something. What is the main cause of skin cancer?

If you are like most people, you probably answered, "the sun."

But if that's the case, then why have the rates of skin cancer increased dramatically just in the last 30 years? Is it because the sun has suddenly changed? Not likely.

As you will soon see, the rise in skin cancer has a LOT more to do with changes in our diet than it does with the sun. If you eat the right foods (and avoid the wrong ones), exposure to the sun will do nothing but improve your health.

Here's something else this book will teach you. The two most common skin cancers – basal cell and squamous cell carcinoma – are easy to treat and rarely fatal. In almost all cases, the cure for them is as simple as having a mole removed. But if you eat like this book suggests and avoid frequent sunburns, you'll never have to worry about it.

So what about melanoma – the deadly form of skin cancer? As you will soon learn the populations that get the LEAST melanoma are those that spend the MOST time in the sun. In other words, office workers have a much higher incidence of melanoma than lifeguards or construction workers. Laboratory studies also show that vitamin D kills melanoma cells – which would explain why melanoma patients have a greater rate of recovery when they spend time in the sun.

If these statements come as a surprise or maybe even a shock to you, don't feel like you're alone. The vast majority of Americans have the same set of erroneous beliefs. For more than thirty years, the sun lotion industry (a $5 billion business) has been supporting the view that the sun is deadly and that we must be protected from it by slavering on chemical compounds.

But the truth is that chemical sunscreens contain as many as five known carcinogens, two of which are actually activated by the sun! And anything above an SPF of 8 blocks your vitamin D production by more than 95%. Quite simply, vitamin D is your best defense against cancer.

The bottom line is this: just about everything the government and mainstream medicine has been telling you about the sun is wrong. Their prescription – stay out of the sun as much as possible and wear sunscreen when you do venture outside – is not only wrong, it's deadly.

In the pages that follow you will get a Masters degree on vitamin D and the sun. You will discover that...

- Our natural environment is the outdoors. Since the beginning of time until only recently we have lived and worked in harmony with the sun. The move from outdoor to indoor living began with the invention of the light bulb in 1879. It was soon after that cancer, heart disease and other degenerative diseases (that our ancestors never experienced) became prevalent.

- Three years ago Dr. Michael Holick, a well-respected chief of endocrinology, nutrition and diabetes at Boston University Medical Center published a book on his research into Vitamin D called The UV Advantage. In that publication he urged people to get enough sunlight to make vitamin D. While many in the medical establishment pilloried his book, hundreds of studies have confirmed Holick's findings.

- Vitamin D modulates the expression of your genes. For example, it regulates the gene that produces C-reactive protein (CRP), that's been linked to heart disease and arthritis. It turns on the gene that produces insulin to control blood sugar. It turns off the gene that produces a certain protein that raises blood pressure dangerously. It increases the production of the enzyme you need to sharpen your thinking and repairs cells that are in danger of causing breast and/or prostate cancer.

- You can't get enough Vitamin D by taking multivitamins. The government recommends 200 to 400 units, depending on your age. But, according to a 2003 study published in the American Journal of Clinical Nutrition, your body needs 2,000 to 5,000 units a day to maintain optimal health (and much more than that when it's stressed). The most reliable way to get what you need is to expose your body to sun.

- There is a good chance your doctor doesn't know about this research. Often, doctors are updated on research by the drug companies, and the drug companies push what is profitable. Inexpensive vitamins and free sunlight are not profitable.

- In the February 2, 2005 issue of the Journal of the National Cancer Institute, a study confirmed that exposure to the sun reduces the risk of skin cancer. Additional studies have shown that lifeguards in Australia have the lowest rates of melanoma. The group that had the highest incidence was office workers.

- A recent study by the National Cancer Institute reveals women whose jobs require consistent sun exposure are much less likely to die of breast cancer.

- Studies also show that men with high exposure to the sun have half the risk of prostate cancer.

- A 1989 study published in the Lancet demonstrated that colon cancer is less prominent among people with regular exposure to the sun.

When I was a kid everyone knew that the sun was good for you. Today – thanks to the Medical-Industrial-governmental complex – we have been scared to death about it. If you want to make your own decision about how much sun you need (and how to get it safely and efficiently), enjoy the pages that follow.

To Your Health,

Michael Masterson

INTRODUCTION

After Decades in the Dark...
It's Time to Reenter Our Native Light

You've been told to avoid sunlight... keep indoors during peak sun hours... cover yourself with sunscreen if you go outside... wear long-sleeved shirts and sunglasses even when it's not sunny... and limit your direct contact with the sun's rays to none.

It may surprise you to learn that any evidence that exposing yourself to the sun is harmful evaporates under scrutiny. It's nothing more than conjecture and slivers of evidence blown out of proportion for commercial interests. What's worse; if you follow this "no safe level of sun exposure" dogma, you'll put yourself at greater risk of numerous deadly cancers, depression, bone loss, heart disease, diabetes and more.

It's time to relearn what we instinctively knew for generations. There is no reason you shouldn't enjoy the warm, golden, mood-lifting rays of the sun. You can and should reap the many health benefits of the sun for a happier and more energetic life.

Just Step Outside and Feel the Benefit

Have you ever noticed how you feel happier sitting or walking in the sun? Doesn't just going outside on a sunny day calm your nerves and lift your spirits?

There's a reason for this. Your body needs sunlight like it needs nutrients. In addition to the noticeable lift it gives your mood, it also helps lower blood pressure, cholesterol and blood sugar, improve immunity, regulate your weight, reverse many chronic diseases, protect you from many cancers and improve your overall health and happiness.

Maybe you're thinking that the sun causes skin cancer... so how can it be healthy? As you will see, this public scare furthers commercialism more than public health. You'll also see why you shouldn't let these commercials disguised as science scare you away from your natural connection with the sun, because sunlight is critical to good health.

Or maybe you're concerned about the increased wrinkling of your skin if you expose it to the sun. As with many other nutrients, you can get too much sun, but that doesn't mean you should avoid it altogether. You will learn simple strategies to prevent wrinkling with normal sun exposure while still enjoying the myriad of health benefits from our most fundamental source of energy, our native sun.

We humans have lived, worked and played in the sun for millennia. Sunlight is as natural to your body as breathing. As with oxygen, if you go without sunlight for long enough, your body suffers. The damage of living without your native sun is more gradual, but in the end, just as deadly.

We Are Born with a Need for Vitamin Sunshine

Sun exposure produces one of the most potent health-boosting substances in your body. This amazing vitamin performs countless valuable functions for you. It can:

- Elevate your mood and boost your mental performance.
- Prevent many types of cancers including prostate, breast and ovarian.

- Reduce your risk of melanoma, the deadly form of skin cancer.
- Prevent and treat the bone diseases of rickets, osteomalacia and osteoporosis.
- Prevent depression and schizophrenia.
- Enhance the function of your pancreas.
- Increase insulin sensitivity and prevent diabetes.
- Help you lose weight.
- Make you sleep better.
- Give you more energy and stamina during the day.
- Significantly lower elevated blood pressure.
- Lower abnormally high blood sugar.
- Decrease bad cholesterol in your blood.
- Increase lymphocytic white blood cells responsible for immunity.

This may be the single most important organic nutrient for your overall health. In fact, if this were a drug, it would be considered the discovery of the century.

This amazingly beneficial nutrient is vitamin D. And we can all get plenty of it free, just by spending enough time in the sun.

How is the Crisis of Vitamin D Deficiency Affecting You?

We are designed, cell by cell, as creatures of the sun. Virtually every organ system in your body is dependent on sunshine for optimal performance. Sunlight triggers vitamin D production in your cells and Vitamin D is an *essential* vitamin. In nutrition, *essential* means that your body cannot function properly without it. It's not widely discussed but your body is literally a living photocell because it draws the energy for this vitamin production from the sun's light.

Over time, adequate sunlight is just as important as air, water, food, rest and sleep. You can only go without air for a few minutes, only go without water for a few days, without food for several weeks before your life will expire. Sunlight starvation won't kill you so quickly, but it can kill you nonetheless.

Epidemics of modern diseases usually result from changes in our environment causing us to live in an unnatural way. Unrecognized when the unnatural change is adopted, the health consequences present themselves later. Whether it's eating processed food our bodies aren't meant to deal with, choosing an unnaturally sedentary lifestyle, or avoiding the sun. These are unnatural choices and they lead to health problems.

Vitamin D deficiency is a very widespread cause of death in the US and Europe. The overall toll that vitamin D deficiency takes has gone unrecognized until recently, but it's immense. This deficiency contributes to the most costly and deadly diseases we face. We would save hundreds of thousands of lives every year if we simply return to spending more time in the sun.

In this book, you will discover how vitamin D helps to prevent internal cancers – deadly cancers like colon, breast, prostate and ovarian cancer. These kinds of cancers and others like them take more than half a million lives every year. Yet, with enough vitamin D, these cancer rates fall dramatically.

You'll also learn the link between depriving yourself of sunlight and your risk of heart disease. Heart disease is the number one killer in the U.S. Vitamin D helps prevent it. And these are just the tip of the iceberg. You'll learn the critical role vitamin D plays in preventing the most feared diseases facing our society.

Put the Power in Your Hands

This idea of sunshine as a vital nutrient may seem novel to you. After all, you've heard so many claims that sunlight is hazardous to your health. Major financial interests have all but squelched the idea of healthy sun exposure.

They tell you to avoid the sun and seek cover. This book includes more than 200 scientific citations exposing this as one of the biggest health blunders of the last fifty years… and, that you sacrifice your health by avoiding the sun.

You don't hear this side of the sun story because nobody makes money when you walk out and get some sunlight on your skin. They can't restrict the sun and sell it back to you in pills. If they could, the sun would be the number one selling drug in the country.

Put aside what you have been told you and take an honest look at the facts about sunlight, vitamin D and health. You'll be surprised at the damage that living in the "dark" does to your body. And you'll uncover the definite good that sunlight does for you.

- You'll find out how sun exposure prevents and treats some of the deadliest cancers like prostate and breast cancers.
- You'll learn how sunlight helps you build strong healthy bones and protects you from osteoporosis.
- You'll discover the role sunshine plays in keeping your heart strong and healthy.
- You'll uncover the answers you need about the sun and skin cancer.
- You'll find step-by-step, actionable advice on how you can benefit from the sun.
- You'll discover how to protect your skin from premature aging and keep your skin looking young and vibrant.

- Plus, you'll discover the foods and supplements to keep your vitamin D levels at their best even when the sun isn't enough.

Best of all, the advice you'll find in this book is easy to understand, inexpensive and simple to put into practice right away.

Now you can begin putting the health benefits of safe sunlight to work in your life.

Start today!

CHAPTER ONE

Farewell Old Friend

How We Came to Abandon Thousands of Years of Experience... and Common Sense

"The sun is the healer, the life-giver. He is the only true doctor to the troubled mind. He is the best apothecary in the world. There is no tonic sold for gold over any chemist's counter so remedial as that celestial pick-me-up which is poured for nothing each morning over the wide counter which is the rim of the earth."

– Norman Davey

The warm rays of the sun are one of life's greatest pleasures. The sun gives you strength and lifts your spirits. As our source of light, warmth, and energy, all life depends on it.

Humans have long celebrated the benefit of the sun through music, art, poetry, and literature. It's one of our universal symbols of happiness. We all seem to be born with an intuitive attraction. Just look through the untainted eyes of a child. At the top of a child's first drawing of his own family or house, you'll usually see a smiling sun.

Yet it's more than a feeling. You have an actual physical need for sunlight for good health. Somehow, people seem to know it. You've probably felt a certain sense of satiation on the first warm day of spring, heading outside to a trail or park. During the winter, thousands of people vacation in warm, sunny climates or ski the slopes where they can bathe in reflected sunshine from the snow-covered hills.

The elderly instinctively migrate south for the winter. The fastest-growing retirement meccas in the United States are in the sunshine-rich southeast and southwest. As you will soon learn, the elderly have a compelling metabolic reason to seek out the sun. The need for sunshine soars in your senior years.

By contrast, consider what happens during the winter months. Many people experience darker moods. As many as 15 million people – possibly more – suffer from a clinical condition called Seasonal Affective Disorder (SAD).[1] You're more likely to get sick during the winter months. You're more likely to gain weight. Come spring, most these symptoms magically evaporate without treatment.

Don't Lock Yourself Away in the Dark

Does it make sense that something that feels so good, that lifts our spirits, and to which we are instinctively drawn, is going to kill us? Of course not. But that's exactly what we're being told by much of the medical establishment, the dermatology profession, and certain corporations with a vested interest.

Every year, these groups spend millions of dollars to promote the belief that sunlight in any amount is dangerous – even deadly. Millions more are spent to promote their products and services. But to convince you that you need them, they must first convince you that your native sun is dangerous.

You'll see that this marketing campaign has distorted the facts about the sun. This book will show you that stern warnings to avoid the sun have contributed to a sharp and steady decline in public health. You'll also find compelling evidence that thousands of people die each year in part because of their separation from sunlight – adding up to millions in the last 3 decades.

How could we have bought into such a colossal mistake?

Throughout History, People Soaked in the Healing Rays of the Sun... Why Not You?

Our ancestors lived in harmony with the sun for hundreds of thousands of years. They lived outdoors every moment of their lives. They hunted for meat, fish and fowl. They spent hours during the day gathering edible plants, fruits and berries from their outdoor surroundings. Later in our history, they planted crops in the open sun.

They ate, worked, gathered, celebrated, worshiped and mourned under the sun.

It was only very, very recently in our history – in the later 19th century – that Thomas Edison brought the commercial light bulb to the market and we had an artificial way to radiate light other than the sun.

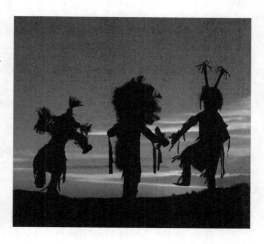

By the 1920s, with the Industrial Revolution well underway, people started migrating from the countryside to find opportunity in the cities. They began working indoors. The average person's standard of living improved greatly with industrialization and specialization of labor.

But unappreciated at the time, this migration indoors altered our ancient relationship with the sun. There is now overwhelming scientific proof that the sun plays a vital role in keeping your body strong, healthy, and free from disease. Our history married us to the sun. In fact, your very physiology – your tissues, cells, organs, and bones and the chemical processes that sustain them – relies upon sunlight.

The average lifespan has dramatically increased in our modern era because of advances in nutrition, sanitation, and medicine, but in many other ways, people were healthier before progress brought us indoors.

While the world around you may have changed, your genetics haven't. You still need sunlight for both optimal health and disease prevention.

A Sudden Change in an Ancient Relationship

For 97 percent of the time that we have lived on this planet, we lived naked in the sun, near the equator.

In evolutionary terms, the shift to indoor living represents a very sudden, recent change. To put this in perspective, imagine the period of our time on earth represented as a single day.

- Only in the last day did we migrate away from the equator.
- Only in the last several hours did we put on clothes.
- Only in the last several minutes did we start working inside.
- Only in the last minute did we start traveling in enclosed vehicles.
- And only in the last second did we cover ourselves in sunscreen.

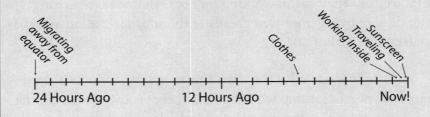

Farewell Old Friend

Less Sunlight Means More Disease

Throughout most of human existence, infectious disease was the number one cause of death. Bacteria, viruses and parasites plagued both young and old. Four out of five children never made it to adulthood. Advances in sanitation and medicine have turned the tables on most infectious diseases.

Now our primary struggle has shifted to degenerative diseases that our ancestors very rarely faced. Heart disease, cancer, diabetes, hypertension, and degenerative neurological problems are commonplace, while they were a rarity just a century ago. And, despite today's avoid-the-sun mentality, we now face a ballooning epidemic of skin cancer.

Our changing relationship with the sun isn't *solely* responsible for the increases in all of these diseases. Chemicals pollute the food you eat, the air you breathe, and the water you drink. You likely eat processed foods made with artificial ingredients and stripped of their nutritional value. Many of the fruits and vegetables you eat contain pesticides and herbicides. The meat you eat probably contains hormones and antibiotics. In place of the daily exertion for survival of your ancestors, most people have adopted a largely sedentary lifestyle, traveling in cars and sitting much of the day.

By altering many of the natural processes that defined our lives for millennia, we've created new health disasters.

MAJOR LIFESTYLE CHANGES IN THE LAST CENTURY	
Then	***Now***
We ate natural, whole foods.	We eat processed foods with chemical preservatives and chemical additives.
We engaged in physical activity often by hunting, foraging, and farming.	Exercise is something we have to *add* to our daily routines.
We spent much of our time outside.	We spend all day indoors.
There was no air or water pollution.	Our water and air contain many carcinogens.

All these changes come with a high price. Declining sun exposure carries its own heavy toll. When you live and work indoors and use sunscreen when you venture out, your levels of vitamin D, the "sunshine vitamin," become too low.

Studies show that a widespread deficiency of vitamin D is rampant in America today and that the average person today has lower vitamin D levels than their parents had just 30 years ago.

There's a link between low sunlight exposure and vitamin D deficiency. There's also a link between low vitamin D levels and other diseases. Research shows that vitamin D reduces the risk of the three biggest killers of our generation – heart disease, cancer, and diabetes.

The Real Connection between Sunlight and Cancer

Most everyone has heard from a family doctor or dermatologist that sun exposure is dangerous. They do have a reason for telling you so.

Over-exposure to the sun – the kind that results in a sunburn – does cause skin damage. It can lead to two types of superficial skin cancer. These kinds of skin cancer, called basal cell and squamous cell, rarely spread to other parts of the body and they are easy to treat. The link between over-exposure to the sun and these kinds of cancer is strong.

However, sun exposure *does not* cause the most deadly form of skin cancer – melanoma. In fact, it has clearly been shown to prevent this form of cancer and to aid in its recovery.

This book will clarify the benefits and dangers of sunlight, and teach you how to get the right amount of sun exposure to be at your healthiest. But before we can truly know our current predicament, we need to explore our forgotten historical relationship with the sun.

Ancient Appreciation of the Therapeutic Affect of the Sun

With instinct as their guide, the ancient Babylonians and Egyptians, Greeks and Romans, the Aztecs, Mayans, and Incas, and the early Chinese, Japanese, and Indian cultures all thought of the sun as the source of health.

"The funeral coach turns twice as often on the shady side of the street." – German Proverb

"Where the sun does not go, the doctor does." – Italian Proverb

They used sunlight as medicine. Ancient cultures used the sun to:

- **Heal their sick children** – Stone plates from Egypt depict the Pharaoh Amenhotep and his wife Nefertiti healing their children of rickets by exposing them to the sun. Many centuries later, certain Germanic tribes placed their feverish children on rooftops.

- **Improve athletic performance** – The Romans believed that "the sun feeds the muscles." They made use of sunlight to strengthen their gladiators. In Greece, the ancient Olympic athletes were also required to take sunbaths.

- **Stop epidemics of disease** – The Romans called upon the God of the Sun, Apollo, to quell an epidemic. In the old epic poem, the *Edda*, you can read about Germans carrying their sick to the mountain slopes to expose them to sunshine.

- **Restore health and prevent illness** – In Greece, Hippocrates – the Father of Medicine – wrote extensively about the healing properties of the sun. The Egyptians erected a city called Heliopolis (City of the Sun) and constructed healing temples where the sick could seek sun therapy. The Romans built solariums for the same purpose.

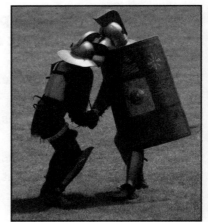

But this knowledge of the sun didn't last. With the fall of the Roman Empire, the Christian church displaced pagan worship. The early Christians stamped out "sun worship" in all its forms, including sunbathing and the use of sunlight in healing. For more than a thousand years, the science of heliotherapy went neglected.

The Rediscovery of Sunlight as Medicine

In the 19th and early 20th centuries, the healing power of sunlight came back into the spotlight. This scientific revolution brought a new way of thinking. Scientists began to study and record the empirical evidence of the benefits of sun exposure.

Despite centuries of "darkness," new science began to observe the health benefits of sunlight. They noticed that some of the healthiest people spent time in the sun. What's more, they discovered that sunlight cured many diseases when nothing else could.

Researchers and scientists made hundreds of important discoveries (and rediscoveries) about sunlight, health, and the formation of vitamin D. In fact, three of these discoveries merited Nobel Prizes. In an era we call the Sunlight Renaissance, scientists around the world reawakened to the healing powers of the sun. Here are just a few of the more important milestones of this period.

THE SUNLIGHT RENAISSANCE

1840

Sunshine Treats Tuberculosis (TB) – 20 percent of the British population suffered from deadly tuberculosis. Dr. George Bodington found that TB was more common in those who spent most of their time indoors. Bodington successfully treated many TB cases by exposing his patients to fresh air and sunlight.

1854

Sunshine Improves Survival in Hospitals – When Florence Nightingale began treating soldiers of the Crimean War, an injured soldier was seven times more likely to die from disease in the hospital than on the battlefield. Nightingale recognized the curative and disinfectant powers of sunlight and insisted that the sun shine into the hospitals. With this and better hygiene, she reduced the death rate in hospitals from 60 percent to 2.2 percent.

1877

Sunshine Kills Bacteria – British researchers Dr. Arthur Downes and Thomas Blunt discovered that sunlight kills harmful microorganisms. They filled test tubes with culture media and left them in a windowsill. The found that the tubes exposed to sunlight remained clear while those in the shade grew cloudy and filled with bacteria. This discovery led to successful sun treatments for bacterial infections.

1882	
Long, Dark Winters Increase Disease – Danish physician Dr. Niels Ryberg Finsen became interested in the study of light when he noticed the negative health effect that the long, dark winters of Denmark had on himself and others.	
UV Lamps Cure TB of the Skin – Dr. Finsen experimented with UV lamps and found they could restore health. He used lamps to cure 98 percent of his patients with TB of the skin (Lupus vulgaris).	

1890	
Sunlight Kills the Bacteria that Cause Tuberculosis – Dr. Robert Koch proved that sunlight actually destroys the bacteria that cause TB.	
Lack of Sunlight Found to Cause Rickets – Observing that urban and northern children had a higher incidence of rickets than children living in the country. T.A. Palm developed his theory about the relationship between rickets and the amount of sunlight in the region. He published his work in the scientific literature.	

1903	
Nobel Prize Awarded for the UV Light Therapy – Dr. Niels Ryberg Finsen won the Nobel Prize for his use of UV light in medicine. In his writings, he made it clear that he preferred to use the sun. He was not the first physician to use light as a medicine, but he was the first to scientifically prove its effects.	
The First Heliotherapy Medical Practice – Dr. Auguste Rollier opened the first heliotherapy clinic (exposing patients to controlled amounts of sunlight) in the Swiss Alps. Rollier's treatment involved prolonged rest, a healthy diet, fresh air, light exercise, and very gradual exposure to sunlight over a period of weeks. His therapy improved the condition of more than 90 percent of his patients.	

1905	
Second Nobel Prize for Study of Sunlight – Dr. Robert Koch won a Nobel Prize for his discoveries that light destroys bacteria and hinders the infection rate.	

1919	
Light Used to Cure Rickets in Children – Dr. Kurt Huldschinsky cured children of rickets by using artificial light. Two years later, researchers at Columbia University proved that sunlight could do the same thing.	

Farewell Old Friend

Cod Liver Oil Eliminates Rickets – At the very same time, British physician Sir Edward Mellanby investigated dietary deficiency in rickets. Testing his theories on dogs, he discovered that cod liver oil (a potent source of vitamin D) cured the condition. Soon after, he used cod liver oil to eliminate rickets in children.

The Discovery of Vitamin D – Nutritional biochemist Elmer McCollum of Johns Hopkins University knew that scientists thought that the vitamin A in cod liver oil was responsible for healing rickets. However, when he destroyed the vitamin A in it, the cod liver oil had the same effect. McCollum then identified the substance that was actually responsible and called it vitamin D.

1928

Nobel Prize Awarded for Uncovering the Structure of Vitamin D – *Adolf Windaus, an organic chemist from Germany, received the Nobel Prize for demonstrating that vitamin D is actually a steroid hormone formed from cholesterol in the body.*

1930

Tens of Thousands Treated with Sunshine – From his first heliotherapy clinic in the Swiss Alps, Dr. Rollier expanded to 36 clinics all over the world with more than 1,000 beds. He successfully cured health conditions ranging from cancer to hypertension, rheumatoid arthritis, rickets, tuberculosis, and bacterial infections. Rollier published a book on the subject: *La Cure de Soleil – Curing with the Sun*.

1933

165 Conditions Treated with UV Light – F.H. Krudsen wrote the book *Light Therapy*, listing 165 conditions that doctors had successfully treated with UV light. Sunbathing grew in popularity and sun therapy was popularized in magazine articles like "The Sun Cure" and "The Miracle of Sunshine." [2]

Synthetic Vitamin D Created – Researchers discovered how to create synthetic vitamin D by irradiating a plant substance known as ergosterol. Soon after, doctors stopped using sunlight to cure rickets.

1937

Researchers Discover Sun Connection to Vitamin D – Nine years after winning the Nobel Prize, Adolf Windaus discovered how vitamin D forms with exposure to UV light. Scientists finally understood how UV light can have the same effect as ingesting vitamin D.

The Birth of Modern Medicine & the Demise of Sunlight

By the 1930s, doctors used light to successfully treat dozens of health conditions. Public service notices encouraged sun exposure as a public health measure. People everywhere once again accepted the healing benefits of the sun. The therapeutic uses of light discovered thousands of years ago and then forgotten had resurfaced.

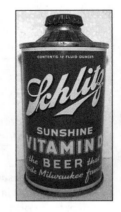

But then the tide began to turn again. In the 1930s, scientists discovered a way to artificially manufacture vitamin D. Soon thereafter, doctors began using synthetic vitamin D to treat rickets. Manufactured vitamin D was more profitable than sunlight and it soon found its way into all manner of consumer products – including beer.

Say Goodbye to Nature – Hello to Pills

During World War I, doctors used sunlight successfully and extensively to treat wounds and infections. But the era of pharmaceuticals began in 1928 with the discovery of penicillin by Sir Alexander Fleming. For the first time in history, drugs could provide a rapid cure for infectious disease.

In 1939, chemist Gerhard Domagk won the Nobel Prize for treating bacterial infections with the antibiotic sulfanilamide and antibiotics soon became the preferred treatment. The advent of the exceptionally profitable pharmaceutical industry spelled the end of sun therapy.

With considerable influence from the new drug industry, doctors soon embraced this view of science and came to believe that we now had the capacity to improve on nature. Doctors began to view natural cures as relics of history.

Another blow to sun therapy occurred in 1941, when *Ladies' Home Journal* published an article where Dr. James Ewing dismissed the benefits of sunlight. He thought that the sun's healing effects really came from outdoor breezes and a general state of relaxation.[3]

In 1959 the American Medical Association declared that sunlight increased skin cancer incidence. From then on, medical professionals said almost nothing good about the sun.

In a few short decades, our perception of the sun changed from miracle healer to predatory menace. Scientists, physicians, and journalists focused entirely on risks, completely forgetting the well-documented benefits. Before long, very few remembered what we once knew about the sun. The consensus became nearly universal that sunlight is a dangerous killer.

Science sometimes dismisses observations if it can't explain the why or how. This was certainly the case with sun therapy. We knew that the sun could alleviate many health conditions, but we couldn't explain how. When it we found that there could be a downside to sun exposure, it became scientifically easier to discount the practice altogether.

How to Undo the Biggest Health Mistake of the Last 50 Years

Today, most of the medical establishment still dismisses the benefits of sunlight (if they are even aware that such benefits exist). We hear often that there's no such thing as a healthy tan. There's an unbalanced emphasis on the hazards of the sun.

As with almost all things in biology, both too little and too much is bad. It should come as no surprise that this is the case with sun exposure. Too much exposure can lead to sunburn and premature aging and can cause certain kinds of skin cancer. But you are likely in for a surprise when it comes to the sun and skin cancer deaths. The sun is definitely not to blame for the increasing death rate from skin cancer. In fact, you'll soon learn that sunlight actually prevents the most deadly forms of skin cancer.

Modern science is now confirming what our primitive ancestors always knew – that the sun is crucial to our physical and mental health. In recent years, numerous respected researchers from some of the most prestigious institutions confirmed that the sun is powerful medicine. There are thousands of studies to support their case. These visionary doctors and scientists clearly prove that our separation from sunlight has been a huge mistake.

In fact, the most serious diseases we currently face are precisely those that sun exposure can help prevent. Its time to reevaluate your relationship with the sun.

Take Your First Step Now for Better Mood, Energy and Health

You can begin to rebuild your own relationship with the sun starting today. Start out slowly with these two simple steps.

Step One: Check your local paper for the sunrise and sunset times in your area. Make it a point to sit quietly and enjoy one or the other. Your ancestors used to get up with the sun, work during the light, and then rest and spend time together once the sun set. You don't have to change the pace of your day to match the sun, but try taking note of its daily cycle. This step will help you feel more in tune with the day and add enjoyment and appreciation to your day, as well.

Step Two: Start reacquainting your skin with the sun. In the morning, before the sun is too high in the sky, go for a short walk outside. Don't put on sunscreen. Don't wear sunglasses. Just walk briefly in the gentle warmth and light of the morning sun for 10 minutes or so.

(Endnotes)

1 "Seasonal Affective Disorder and Light Therapy," Information provided by the Cleveland Clinic Health Information Center. 8/18/2006

2 Lillyquist, MJ. *Sunlight and Health: The Positive and Negative Effects of the Sun on You.* New York: Dodd Mead and Company. p. 24

3 Lillyquist, MJ. *Sunlight and Health: The Positive and Negative Effects of the Sun on You.* New York: Dodd Mead and Company. p. 35

CHAPTER TWO

Sun Police Put Your Health at Risk

"Dermatologists tell you to hide from the sun and modern living would lead us to believe we can do just fine by living in caves – offices, homes, and automobiles. But our genetic roots tell us we should be naked and in a climate where we can be so. That is our origin – and what was the norm for 99.99% of our history. Should we believe dermatologists and modern lifestyle or our genes and history?"

– Dr. Randy Wysong

For all but the smallest, most recent part of our history, we've lived in harmony with the sun. Our ancestors worshipped it as the source of life. The earliest physicians swore by its healing powers. Even just two generations ago, the medical profession and health authorities praised the benefits of sun exposure.

In this book, you'll learn that sunlight really is everything our ancestors knew it to be – a powerful healing force essential for optimal health. Yet like most things in life, sunlight is good for you in the right doses and too much can be harmful.

The sun can lift your spirits and boost your energy, but too much sun will sap your strength. Science shows that the sun can dramatically boost your immunity, but too much will weaken it. Likewise, moderate and sensible sun exposure will give you a light, healthy tan and provide tremendous benefits to your overall health.

But too much sunlight will burn and blister your skin, leading to premature aging and, potentially, the superficial skin cancers.

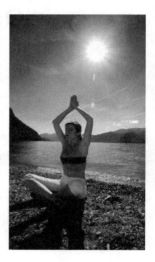

The same is true of exercise. You know that exercise can boost your energy, raise your immunity, and improve your health. But too much exercise can wear down your body, deplete your immune system, and damage your health.

The enjoyment of food is healthy. Gluttony is not. Wine is good for you. Alcoholism is not. As with nearly every-thing in life, moderation should be your guide when it comes to enjoying the rays of the sun.

Unfortunately, a powerful, vocal minority has a financial stake in a one-sided outcome of this debate. For this group, a simple re-turn to moderation and common sense leaves them without a job. Their mission is to drown out any discussion of the issue. They even claim that those who advocate moderate sun exposure threaten public health.

In this chapter, you'll see for yourself, the questionable motives of the "sun police" and why they've created a climate of fear and sought to squelch dissent.

Why Commercialism Benefits from Fear of the Natural

When financial incentives become mixed with emerging medical science, their influence can be surprisingly successful at distorting the public perception of what the science really proves.

Witness the success of the large grain packagers at convincing an entire nation to radically change what we ate for breakfast for generations.

When a corporation can turn 4 cents worth of wheat or corn into a four dollar box of cereal, it pays for a lot of promotional effort. But you can't mark up an egg very much because anyone else can sell the same product. Unlike our natural diet, processed products are proprietary, that is, no one else can sell your brand of artificial, processed food, which allows for higher margins. This extreme marketing advantage for artificial products has resulted in a multimedia deluge of the supposed health advantages of a new pure carbohydrate processed grain breakfast. But their success was also incumbent on first convincing us that our traditional breakfast was somehow unsafe.

Only recently has the public begun to have an appreciation of the real science that had been unchampioned, but present, all along. That is that our ancestral custom of a high protein breakfast had developed and persisted for so long for good reason. Eggs are loaded with vitamins and amino acids that get into your blood unusually fast in the morning and charge you up for the day. The truth is that eating eggs was never and is still not linked to heart disease. Yet the cholesterol issue has successfully served as a convenient red herring to launch the most profitable food category in history.

This is not to suggest that these things are planned conspiracies. The financial reality alone can insidiously, (and with remarkably low public awareness), drive the outcome.

Sunlight and health is one of many examples where such powerful financial incentives can take a sliver of a medical truth and distort it to suggest something more – something that better promotes the public perception of need for a product.

When the sunscreen industry was born in the 70's, their message was to use their products to prevent sunburn and allow for healthy tanning during rare times of unusually high sun exposure.

When the medical establishment began accumulating evidence that too much sun could be harmful, profits from sunscreens were used to further this message and a new branch

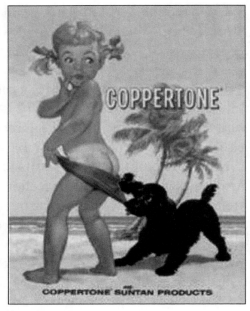

of the skin care industry was born. It soon grew to billions in annual revenues.

These new skincare products served as the financial engine that worked to "raise awareness" about the link between skin cancer and the sun. Every year since that time, these companies spend tens of millions of dollars to perpetuate the belief that sunlight is harmful.

Certainly, too much sunlight can do damage – but we receive nothing but warnings to avoid the sun. There is no corresponding advice about the benefits of sun exposure.

Wouldn't any marketer like to expand the use of their existing products? What if you could change the perception of these products from a rare and specialized need for skiers or summer beach goers to virtually every man, woman and child - every day? Even better, if you could find a related industry that shared your financial interest, you could team up and make your case even more convincing.

Here the industry found a lucky convergence of forces. Medicine was in the midst of the biggest medicalization in its history. That is to say, every societal issue was being converted into a medical one. Enter the dermatological profession. We would all need their services if they could convince us that we were unsafe without their expertise.

Consider this recent quote from Dr. Boni Elewski, president of the American Academy of Dermatology:

> *"Any group, organization, or individual that disseminates information encouraging exposure to UV radiation – whether natural or artificial – is doing a disservice to the public."*

Or just look at these messages taken directly from dermatological websites:

- "Sunlight is dangerous; it can kill you."
- "Sunlight is a known carcinogen – there is NO safe level of exposure."
- "There is no such thing as a healthy tan."
- "Always wear a hat and protective clothing when outside."
- "Wear sunscreen at all times over all exposed areas."

This message is clear enough: Stay out of the sun. If you do venture outdoors, **wear sunscreen** from morning to night, summer and winter, on every exposed inch of skin.

We have all but forgotten that sunscreen-makers originally marketed their products to *promote* tanning while protecting you from sunburn. Now, you should wear sunscreen to *protect* yourself from the sun. This has been a clever and successful shift. You need their products, all the time or you'll get cancer.

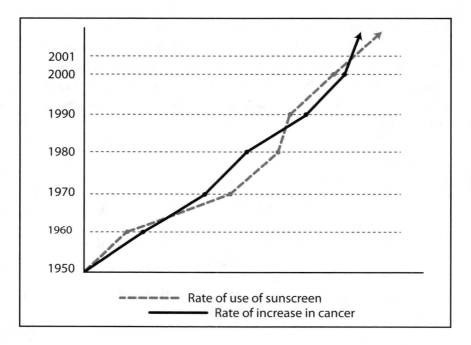

Now for a reality check. Unfortunately, the campaigns sell sunscreen, but they haven't decreased skin cancer—skin cancer rates skyrocketed in the past three decades since sunscreens have become billion dollar products. In fact, in this book you will learn that sunscreen could very well be the primary *cause* of the increase in skin cancer.

In Chapters 5, you will also see that there is more to skin cancer than just sun exposure. And you will learn why *less* sun has resulted in *more* deadly internal cancers.

There's one more problem with the notion that we should ignore human history and strive for less exposure to the sun... and it's a big one.

Finally, Some Light Shines on Vitamin D

Like the resurgence of the lowly egg, a string of recent studies are awakening the medical community to the vital health importance of vitamin D – a substance your body can only produce in abundance with sunlight. (Ironically, the egg was one of your best natural dietary sources of vitamin D before we were convinced that it would kill us.)

The evidence has recently forced even the anti-sun lobby to admit the importance of vitamin D to human health. They are on public record that a vitamin D deficiency is dramatically increasing the risks of several deadly diseases.

Unfortunately, they failed to vindicate themselves for their error and recommend the return to natural sunlight. Instead, they dismiss evolutionary history and our very physiology and insist that the sun is not the best source of vitamin D. But rather, they propose that we meet our need for Vitamin D with pills or foods artificially fortified with vitamin D.

Unfortunately, if you follow this advice and avoid the sun while relying on artificially fortified foods and Vitamin D supplements, you are virtually guaranteed to be deficient in this most important nutrient.

The truth is that very few foods naturally contain our required vitamin D. Those that do provide only a small amount. Fortified foods are worse. To get the bare minimum amount of the vitamin D you need without getting any help from the sun, you would have to drink 30 glasses of fortified milk every day. Even most nutritional supplements do not contain nearly enough vitamin D to ensure optimal health.

Despite all efforts to sell us yet another product, the simple truth remains that *we are designed* to get Vitamin D from the sun, not Vitamin D fortified cow's milk or Flintstone's chewables. Fixing this problem is so vital to your good health that you will find the next two chapters devoted to it alone.

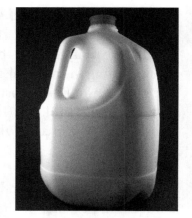

We now live indoors, drive in cars that are covered, and work in buildings under artificial lights. Yet, you still hear that you should avoid the sun and slather your skin with sunscreen when you do venture into daylight.

How did the public health authorities miss the boat and advise us of something so against our nature? You may realize that this is not the first time we've been led astray by new science that seems to suggest we should forget our roots, traditions and even common sense.

Modern Medicine's Track Record of Dangerous Trends

Just look at some of our health belief changes in recent years.

What New Science Claimed Then:	What We Later Learned:
Eggs will kill you with cholesterol so you must change to no-cholesterol cereals.	Eggs are among the healthiest of foods and don't increase risk of heart attack or stroke.

What New Science Claimed Then:	What We Later Learned:
Margarine is a health food.	Artificial margarine promotes inflammation and heart disease.
Vegetable oils are health foods.	Vegetable oils promote inflammation and heart disease.
Baby formula is superior to breast milk.	Breast milk is far superior to any synthetic formula.
If you want to lose weight, eat more low-fat products.	Weight comes off by eating natural fat and avoiding low-fat, high carb products.
Only drugs cure diseases.	Natural nutrients are often the most fundamental cure for disease.

Notice that in each case, there were big profits to be made by believing the supposition on the left, while the later proven view on the right relied on a lower cost, natural solution.

Yet even our most distinguished medical institutions have been wrong in each case. If the past is any indication, it may be years before the majority of medical professionals recognize the necessity of sunlight to your good health.

Remember the example of the lowly egg. Billions were made selling cereal, but first they had to convince you that your traditional breakfast was no longer safe.

Billions to Be Made, but First You Have to Fear Your Native Sun

"Efforts are made in many circles to convince the public that enjoying sunlight is extremely hazardous. Much of this is pretense with a commercial bias."

– Dr. Herbert M. Shelton (1934)

The loudest supporters of sun avoidance directly profit from these views. The "cosmeceutical" industry merges cosmetics and pharmaceuticals. Fear of the sun is an integral part of this business. Market researchers estimate that the cosmeceutical industry sells $30 billion worth of products every year with $6 billion in annual sales of sunscreens alone.

These businesses make billions by emphasizing the harmful effects of sunlight – but no one makes big profits defending the sun. No wonder the spokespeople for this industry have been so successful at drowning out the opposing view. They overstate the risks, deny that there are benefits, and then inundate us with the message that their sunscreen should be worn daily in all climates.

The dermatology profession plays right along. In fact, the American Academy of Dermatology (AAD) is a major force in the anti-sun movement. When you follow the trail of money, you find that the sunscreen industry provides generous funding to the AAD.

By its own admission, the American Academy of Dermatology depends heavily on "corporate partners," stating on its website that "corporate support is vital to the Academy's extensive programs ..." Among the companies that support the AAD, you'll find numerous sunscreen manufacturers along with companies in the business of fortifying foods with vitamin D.[1]

Sun Police Put Your Health at Risk

This financial allegiance to the sunscreen industry unduly influences the AAD. However, this is not the only bias of dermatologists. Most are also susceptible to the phenomenon of over-specialization of their health concern. With their concern focused solely on the skin, they often overlook other biological systems, many of which depend on sunlight.

Don't be Convinced by the Propaganda – Check Facts Yourself

You may be surprised to discover that a similar commercial agenda taints what are called "public service" campaigns. These campaigns seem genuine at first glance. It turns out that most of these groups have direct ties to the cosmeceutical corporations.

Take the Sun Safety Alliance, for instance. This sounds benign enough. It's behind one of the most visible skin cancer prevention campaigns in the US. And, like many of the others, the organization says that even a small amount of sun exposure is unacceptable. They recommend complete abstinence from sun exposure for all ages, in all climates. According to the Alliance:

- You need to apply sunscreen liberally and evenly over all exposed skin.
- Apply a sunscreen with an SPF of 15 or higher whenever you're outdoors.
- Stay in the shade whenever possible.
- Always wear protective clothing when outside.
- Keep babies completely out of the sun.

So what, exactly, is the Sun Safety Alliance? You have to read the fine print to learn that it's a front for "Coppertone Suncare Products and the National Association of Chain Drugstores." Of course, like all companies, their goal is to sell more of their products for bigger profits. Masquerading as an unbiased party with your health as their primary concern may be clever marketing, but you should not mistake their message as science.

The Sun Safety Alliance at Work

The following is a children's media presentation from the Sun Safety Alliance:

"We UV rays got all these powers,
damage can happen in minutes, not hours.
We can burn your skin and you won't even know.
Sometimes you'll turn red, sometimes it won't show.
So you have to be careful when you're out having fun.
Don't let unprotected skin get kissed by the sun.
But don't worry, we'll tell you what you can do
To grow old and be healthy until 102 ...
About a half-hour before you step outside
Is the time that sunscreen should be applied.
Cover all your parts, and have a routine.
And make sure it's at least SPF 15."

The presentation goes on to stress the importance of wearing sunscreen on cloudy days, in winter and even in the car.[2]

Yet much of the real research on sunlight concludes that sun exposure plays a vital role in overall health and longevity. You're just not hearing about it. You don't hear about pro-sun outcomes of research because the voice of the anti-sun lobby is so much better funded it drowns it out.

Unfortunately, the industry has also been able to intimidate those who do try to promote the benefits of sun exposure with deep criticism and even professional consequences.

Consider the case of Dr. Michael Holick.

One Doctor Dared to Speak Out and Lost His Job

*"Science is supposed to be an island of rationality in
a sea of intolerance. Yet intolerance is rearing its ugly
head here as well. Astonishingly, advocating even
a few minutes of exposure to Old Sol these days is
enough to get you blackballed by your profession,
regardless of prior accomplishments."*

– Dr. Ralph Moss, Ph.D. (author of 11 books on cancer research)

Thirty years ago, Dr. Michael Holick, Ph.D., M.D., worked as a graduate student with his professor, Dr. Hector DeLuca and helped discover how vitamin D works in the body. He went on to make many discoveries regarding vitamin D with landmark contributions to our understanding of the human endocrine system.

In 2003, Dr. Holick was a professor of dermatology and the chief of the endocrinology, nutrition, and diabetes department of Boston University Medical Center.[3] That year he authored a book based on his research, *The UV Advantage*, in which he presented a compelling argument for people to get enough sunlight for their bodies to produce vitamin D by spending brief amounts of time in the sun for a few days each week.

When Dr. Holick's book came out, the dermatology profession met it with surprisingly ferocious opposition. As part of the outcry, Dr. Barbara Gilchrest, the current head of the dermatology department at Boston University, called it "an embarrassment" and Dr. Holick was asked to resign his teaching position.

Dr. Holick is a serious and well-credentialed scientist. He has authored more than 200 peer-reviewed studies on the subject of vitamin D since 1970, while his most vocal critics haven't authored a single paper on the subject.

Dr. Holick didn't advocate prolonged exposure to the sun. He advised common sense and suggested people simply spend a few minutes in the sun a few days a week. Despite his impeccable scientific background and the wealth of research he had done proving his position, the dermatology profession immediately ostracized him.

Just how have the policymakers arrived at the conclusion that sensible sun exposure is so damaging to human health? After all, the American Academy of Dermatology still proclaims that there is NO safe level of sun exposure, and the U.S. government lists sunlight as a known carcinogen.

The studies used to back these claims are lacking, to put it mildly. There simply are none that prove that normal, moderate sun exposure has damaging effects on our skin!

Scientific studies are most conclusive when they isolate a single variable. To conduct controlled research on the effects of moderate sun exposure on the human body, researchers would need two groups of people with matched ages, genders, states of health, diets, lifestyles, and environmental conditions. The primary variable would need to be the amount of sunlight that each group received.

To date this kind of research has never been done. Such research simply isn't available. Other studies have been used, but they are far from clinical proofs.

The Tests That the Sunlight Is Dangerous Were Rigged

Dr. Jacob Liberman, O.D., Ph.D., has looked extensively for the existence of such evidence that "proved" the dangers of the sun and concluded that it was completely lacking of any proof that UV light leads to skin cancer or causes damage to our vision:

- **Sunlight and Eye Damage** – One study that received a good deal of attention by the sunglass industry took place in 1981 at the Medical College of Virginia. In this experiment, scientists tranquilized a group of monkeys. They chemically dilated the monkeys' eyes so their pupils would remain wide open. Then they pried their eyes open with clamps and beamed a 2500-watt xenon light into them for 16 minutes.[4] This study showed that the monkeys suffered retinal damage. In case you were planning on doing that to yourself, now you know not to.

- **Sunlight and Skin Cancer** – An equally misinterpreted series of studies form the basis for reports that the sun causes skin cancer. In these tests, scientists repeatedly burned the skin of rabbits and hairless mice with high-intensity UV light. The animals developed skin cancer.[5]

These experiments simply don't simulate the native environment necessary for a valid test. And they certainly do not form a basis for credible scientific conclusions. Rabbits and mice normally have hair to protect them from overexposure to the sun. Neither you nor a monkey would stare directly into the sun for 16 minutes. In normal circumstances the pupils of a monkey's eyes, when exposed to bright sunlight, would naturally constrict to protect his retina ... as would yours.

Yet sunscreen purveyors used these studies to make claims like, "Research indicates that UV light causes skin cancer and eye damage in laboratory animals."

You Deserve a Sensible Alternative

How much ultraviolet light is safe? Now that is a legitimate topic for scientific debate, but we hear only one side of the issue. The side that you don't hear is that ultraviolet sunlight (particularly UVB radiation) isn't always bad for your health.

In *The UV Advantage*, Dr. Holick points out that the attitude of our national health leaders seems to be "We can't trust the public to be judicious in its attitude toward sun exposure, so let's tell them they shouldn't spend any time in the sun." If you think the sun will kill you, you're less likely to overexpose yourself to it. The problem with this approach is that staying completely *out* of the sun can also kill you.

Don't be Swayed by Sun-Paranoia

Your very physiology is designed to harvest sunlight. Moderate exposure is as important to your health as pure water, fresh air, physical activity, and nutritious food. The next few chapters will help you weigh the pros of sun exposure against the cons. Make your own decision. But don't be swayed by corporations that have a vested interest.

The sun police shun any recommendation for moderation. But when it comes to the sun, moderation is essential. Sunlight conveys one of our most precious natural resources – vitamin D. Vitamin D gives you an amazing array of health benefits, including protection against heart disease, diabetes, and deadly internal cancers. Read on to the next chapter for the rest of the story on Vitamin D from sunlight..

(Endnotes)

1 The American Academy of Dermatology. (2006). Corporate Partner Support. http://www.aad.org/aad/support/corporatepartnersupport.htm

2 Moss, EF. (2003). Block the sun, not the fun. The Sun Safety Alliance. http://www.sunsafetyalliance.org/user-assets/Flash/Block_The_Sun_Final.swf

3 The Associated Press. (2005). Vitamin D research may have doctors pre-scribing sunshine. USA Today, May 21, 2005. http://www.usatoday.com/news/nation/2005-05-21-doctors-sunshine-good_x.htm

4 Ham, WT et al. (1982). Action Spectrum for Retinal Injury From Near-Ultravi-olet Radiation in the Aphakik Monkey. *Am J Ophthalmol.* 93(3):299-306.

5 Liberman, J. (1991). *Light: Medicine of the Future.* Rochester, VT: Bear and Company. p. 147

CHAPTER THREE

Reclaim Your Most Ancient Hormone

"Are we supposed to dismiss millions of years
of evolution because "modern" science does not
understand the supreme wisdom of nature?"

– Dr. Jacob Liberman

Most of us wake up in a dark room, travel inside of an enclosed car, put on glasses to block out the light, work all day under artificial lights, and then drive home not long before sunset.

Then when we do go in the sun, we slather on sunscreen. As far as your body is concerned, you're living in darkness.

This is not your genetic heritage. You're designed to live in the sun. Only 100,000 years ago we migrated to climates with less sun, then we began covering our skin. Until most recently, even this was to protect ourselves from the cold of our new environment – not the sun.

More recently, our transportation evolved from horses to cars, further preventing the rays of the sun from reaching us. Finally, only in the last 30 years, we began using sunscreen and avoiding the sun altogether.

How Hiding from the Sun Hurts Your Health

Over the last couple of decades, we've seen the average level of the most potent steroid hormone in the human body fall dramatically. You already know the name of this hormone... it's vitamin D.

If you're deficient in vitamin D, genes designed to protect your health can't work properly, because they need vitamin D to switch them on. One of the most significant scientific discoveries of the century was the role of vitamin D in health maintenance. This discovery alone will have a dramatic impact on disease prevention, including cancer.

Understanding the role of vitamin D is an important key to taking control of your own health. This knowledge will help you see why a balanced and natural relationship with the sun is so important. Right now, if you are like most people, you probably spend at least 90% of daylight hours indoors. We are going to show you why it's important to spend more time in the sun and how you can do this safely.

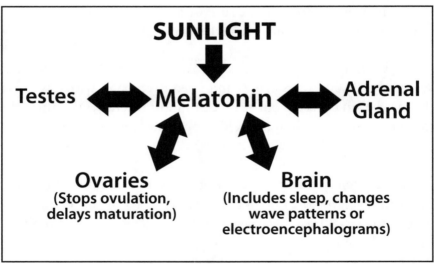

Melatonin affects glands of the body.

Vitamin D Isn't Just a Vitamin

By definition, a "vitamin" is an organic substance that's required by the body, but can't be made by the body. Vitamins must be acquired through the diet. A hormone, on the other hand, is a substance produced by specific organs and carried through the bloodstream affecting other organ systems.

The vitamin D produced in your skin is not technically a hormone, but a pro-hormone. In other words, it provides the raw material from which a hormone is produced. And the hormone that is produced from vitamin D is one of the most important hormones in the human body.

To understand the significance of vitamin D in keeping your body well, it is important to understand how your body makes and uses it.

Understanding How Your Body Makes Vitamin D

Your endocrine system produces vitamin D. The endocrine system is a series of ductless glands that regulate your body's functions by producing hormones and releasing them into the blood stream. The endocrine system creates vitamin D in three steps:

1. Sunlight strikes pre-cholesterol molecules in your skin, transforming them into large quantities of **cholecalciferol** (vitamin D3). This is the naturally occurring form of vitamin D. It can also be taken as a supplement.

2. Your bloodstream absorbs this cholecalciferol and transports it to the liver where it's converted to **calcidiol** (25-hydroxyvitamin D). Although this form of vitamin D doesn't have significant biological activity, it's vital in the next step of the vitamin D process.

3. Calcidiol is then transported to the kidneys first and then to other tissues of the body where it is converted into the potent

steroid hormone **calcitriol** (1,25-dihydroxyvitamin D). It is this form of "activated" vitamin D that goes to work protecting your body from disease.

Here's a flow chart of this process.

Ultraviolet light + pre-cholesterol in the skin	→	cholecalciferol (vitamin D3) + oxygen in the liver	→	calcidiol (25-hydroxyvitamin D... biologically weak) + kidneys/ other tissues	→	calcitriol (1,25-dihydroxy-vitamin D... activated form of vitamin D)

This final form of vitamin D is the most potent steroid hormone in the human body. It's active in amounts as small as one trillionth of a gram. And we are just now beginning to understand how this complex system works.

Your Real Evolutionary Missing Link

Your physiology is as closely linked to the sun as that of plants. Plants use sunlight to photosynthesize chlorophyll. Your body uses a comparable process to photosynthesize vitamin D. Sunlight and vitamin D touch virtually every aspect of your biochemistry and physiology.

In fact, vitamin D is so important to your body, that soon after we began to move away from the equator, some of us began to develop fair skin. With fair skin, we could still synthesize vitamin D with the weaker northern sun. But for even fair-skinned people to produce vitamin D, they must still expose their skin to unblocked sunlight.

Let's look more closely at just a small number of the vital roles that vitamin D plays in your health:

Reclaim Your Most Ancient Hormone

- Autocrine cellular functions – this process occurs within the cells and helps cells to regulate the expression of genes.
- Paracrine cellular functions – this is the process by which cells produce hormones, growth factors and other substances which affect other local cells.
- Regulates and assists in calcium absorption
- Helps to regulate apoptosis (programmed cell death)
- Energy metabolism
- Muscle strength and coordination
- Facilitates neurotransmitter production
- Reduces C-reactive protein (CRP) and other markers of inflammation
- Brain development
- Insulin production stimulation
- Modulates immune system function
- Has an effect on myocardial contractility (helps your heart to beat properly).
- Prevents inflammatory bowel disease
- Inhibits the blood pressure hormone renin

You see how varied the important work that vitamin D does in your body really is. Let's look more closely at two of the biggest benefits of vitamin D – maintaining calcium levels in your blood and preventing disease in your genes.

Build Strong Bones and a Healthy Immune System

One of the primary roles of vitamin D is to maintain normal calcium levels in the blood.

Of course, you know that calcium is essential for the maintenance of bone tissue. What you may not realize is that when it comes to your bones – and more – calcium and vitamin D have a symbiotic relationship. If you're missing either one, the other can't do its job.

Healthy calcium levels are crucial. Calcium controls innumerable processes in your body including responses in your muscles, bones and glands. In addition to its role in bone health, this vital mineral:

- Helps the central nervous system transmit nerve impulses.
- Helps the muscles to contract.
- Influences the secretion of insulin by the pancreas.
- Regulates the immune system.

You get calcium from the food you eat, or from supplements. But your body needs vitamin D in order to absorb calcium (and phosphorous) from the intestinal tract. No matter how much calcium you ingest, without enough vitamin D your body can't absorb it from the small intestine.

Without Vitamin D, You Put Your Cells at High Risk for Cancer

Your body's first priority for calcidiol, the weak form of vitamin D, is to transport it to the kidneys to make calcitriol (activated vitamin D). Activated vitamin D circulating in the blood keeps your blood calcium levels high. Calcium is essential for far more than just bones. Research shows that calcium and vitamin D deficiency in combination puts you at risk for a wide array of chronic diseases.[1]

But your body needs calcidiol for a second vital function. After the kidneys have enough calcidiol, the rest goes directly to your cells, where they convert it to activated vitamin D in a form that your tissues can use. This activated vitamin D goes to work on a cellular level fighting cancer and disease.

Why does this matter? If you are chronically short of calcidiol because you don't get enough sunshine, your tissues won't receive any. Think of it like a gas tank. When you keep your tank full of vitamin D, you ensure that it will flow to every part of the body that needs it. And it appears that the more calcidiol your tissues receive, the more activated vitamin D they will create.

Calcium and vitamin D work together to decrease the risk of malignancies in the colon, breasts and prostate and help prevent a wide range of inflammatory, autoimmune, and metabolic disorders.[2] Studies suggest that 90% of the population is deficient in one,

Lack of Sunlight and Kidney Cancer

Using newly available data on worldwide cancer incidence to map cancer rates in relation to proximity to the equator , researchers a the Moores Cancer Center at University of California San Diego (UCSD) have shown a clear association between deficiency in exposure to sunlight ultraviolet B (UVB) and kidney cancer.

Researchers created a graph with a vertical axis for renal cancer incidence rates, rates and a horizontal axis for latitude. The latitudes range from -90 for the southern hemisphere, to zero for the equator, to +90 for northern hemisphere. Then they spotted incidence rates for 175 countries according to latitude. The resulting chart was a parabolic curve that looks like a smile.

Countries with the highest cancer rates were places like New Zealand and Uruguay in the southern hemisphere and Iceland and the Czech Republic in the northern hemisphere. Clustered at the bottom of the curve with the lowest incidence rates were Guam, Indonesia and other equatorial countries on most continents, including many varied equatorial cultures.

the other, or both.

Vitamin D Helps Prevent Osteoporosis

When your body is short of calcium, it pulls it from your bones. This leads to osteoporosis.

The process works like this. You have a gland called the parathyroid gland. It has a calcium sensor. When your body needs calcium, this gland produces a hormone called PTH which signals the kidneys to make more vitamin D. The circulating vitamin D is what allows the calcium in your diet to be absorbed through the intestines.

Because calcium is so important, if there is not enough calcium in your diet or not enough vitamin D to facilitate its absorption, then vitamin D and the the parathyroid hormone (PTH) will work together to pull this mineral from the bones. The result is osteoporosis.

Ideally, you want to have low levels of PTH, so your body never gets the signal to draw calcium from the bones. To keep your PTH levels low, you need enough calcium in your system. To keep enough calcium in your system, you need enough vitamin D.

You Have Vitamin D Receptors
All Throughout Your Body

Does it seem strange that vitamin D has such a wide range of therapeutic and health-related benefits? The reason is that almost all the cells and tissues in your body have a receptor for vitamin D.

Activated vitamin D is one of the most potent regulators of cell growth in both normal and cancerous cells. It helps to determine

Reclaim Your Most Ancient Hormone

what each cell becomes. As a result, vitamin D can dramatically decrease your risk of cancer.

You see, vitamin D inhibits abnormal cell growth. It also causes cells to mature and die when they are supposed to. When these processes malfunction, cancer can get a foothold in your body. Did you know that people who live at higher latitudes are more prone to developing common cancers and dying of them? The reason is that they are more prone to vitamin D deficiencies.

Colon Cancer and Latitude:

Country:	Latitude (°):	Death Rate Per 100,000 Population:
Northern Ireland	54	16.4
Republic of Ireland	53	16.6
England and Wales	52	15.3
Netherlands	52	14.7
Germany	51	16.5
Belgium	50	15.5
Austria	47	15.2
Switzerland	47	12.2
France	46	11.2
Canada	45	13.5
New Hampshire, USA	44	11.5
New York, USA	43	12.4
Connecticut, USA	42	11.5
Rhode Island, USA	42	12.2
Massachusetts, USA	42	12.1
Italy	42	10.5
New Zealand	41	19.7

New Jersey, USA	40	12.9
Spain	40	7.8
Greece	39	5.2
Japan	36	9.3
New Mexico, USA	34	8.8
Arizona, USA	34	15.8
Israel	31	11.8
Chile	30	6.1
Florida, USA	28	9.9
Mexico	23	2.7
Hawaii, USA	20	8.5
Guatemala	15	0.5

Breast Cancer and Latitude:

Country:	Latitude (°):	Death Rate Per 100,000 Population:
Northern Ireland	54	26.9
Republic of Ireland	53	25.7
England and Wales	52	29.0
Netherlands	52	25.8
Germany	51	21.9
Belgium	50	25.6
Austria	47	22.0
Switzerland	47	24.9
France	46	19.0
Canada	45	23.5
New Hampshire, USA	44	25.0
New York, USA	43	25.6

Reclaim Your Most Ancient Hormone

Connecticut, USA	42	23.6
Rhode Island, USA	42	25.7
Massachusetts, USA	42	25.0
Italy	42	20.4
New Zealand	41	25.0
New Jersey, USA	40	25.8
Spain	40	15.0
Greece	39	15.1
Japan	36	5.8
New Mexico, USA	34	19.4
Arizona, USA	34	20.0
Israel	31	22.5
Chile	30	12.7
Florida, USA	28	20.9
Mexico	23	6.3
Hawaii, USA	20	6.3
Guatemala	15	2.3

Scientists have also found that your body has vitamin D receptor sites throughout all the organs. These receptor sites are genetically designed to bind with activated vitamin D. Think of these receptor sites as puzzle pieces. Without the matching piece of the puzzle – activated vitamin D – they don't fulfill their function of turning genes on and off as the body needs. These genes that normally resist cancer, can actually promote cancer without activated vitamin D.

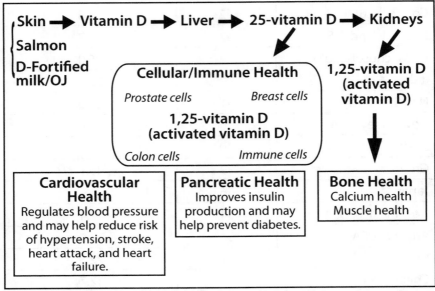

New understanding of how vitamin D benefits health.

The more activated vitamin D your body can create, the better.

Amount of Calcidiol	Course in the body	Result
Severely deficient due to lack of sunshine and subsequent lack of calcidiol.	The body has little calcidiol for the kidney to make *cacitriol* for the blood.	Calcium levels in blood are compromised and virtually no calcidiol gets to the tissues.
More is available, but still deficient.	Virtually all of the calcidiol is still sent to the kidneys to make *cacitriol* in the blood.	The body has enough to maintain calcium levels in the blood; almost none gets to the tissues.

Adequate calcidiol due to sunshine and/or vitamin D supplementation.	After the kidneys have enough, the rest floods directly to cells where *calcitriol* is made for the tissues.	Maintenance of calcium levels AND flooding of receptor sites throughout your body with activated vitamin D.

You should do everything you can to make sure your body has enough activated vitamin D to go around!

If you have sufficient vitamin D to get to your tissues, your cells will convert it to activated vitamin D. The activated vitamin D works inside your cells triggering certain genes to switch on and off. This is important because these genes are either fighting or promoting cancer. In fact, billions of cells use vitamin D to respond to a wide variety of diseases and help the body heal.

Your Whole Body Depends on Vitamin D

In tissues throughout your body, activated vitamin D signals your genes to make hundreds of different enzymes, proteins, hormones and neurontransmitters that are crucial to maintaining health and fighting disease. Tissues in the prostate, breasts, colon, small intestine, bones, immune cells, brain, heart, skin, testicles, and most other organs in the body can activate vitamin D and use it for their specific needs.

In the monthly newsletter produced by the Vitamin D Council, Dr. John Cannell describes five of the many ways activated vitamin D helps you prevent or heal disease through controlling your genes.

Activated Vitamin D – Your Body's Genius Problem Solver

Activated Vitamin D	The Problem	Vitamin D's Solution
Protects you from cardiovascular disease and arthritis	Your body is producing too much of the inflammatory C-reactive protein (CRP)	Turns off the gene that makes CRP
Controls your blood sugar	Your pancreas needs to produce more insulin to control blood sugar	Turns on the gene to make more insulin
Regulates your blood pressure	Your kidney produces too much of a certain protein that raises your blood pressure	Turns off the gene that makes that protein
Helps prevent cloudy thinking and depression	Your brain is not making enough neurotransmitters	Increases production of the enzyme you need to make these neurotransmitters
Helps you prevent cancer	Your breast or prostate begins to develop cancer cells	Forces those cells to remain normal and then die when they are supposed to

The more we learn, the more we understand that activated vitamin D plays a role in virtually every aspect of your health. More than thirty different tissues in the body have receptor sites to collect and use it, including the heart, stomach, pancreas, brain, skin, prostate, colon, breasts, testicles and white blood cells of the immune system (lymphocytes). [3]

Calcitriol is so potent that it is active in minute quantities. Dr. John Cannell tells us in his article "*The Secrets of Vitamin D Production*" that vitamin D becomes active in picogram quantities or 1/1,000,000,000,000 of a gram.[4] It is one of the most potent, powerful nutrients you can give to your body.

Have You Been Tested for Vitamin D Deficiency?

So how much vitamin D do you need to ensure that your kidneys and your tissues receive it? What's the best way to get it? Good questions.

But first, let's look at the best way to determine if you're deficient in vitamin D. Most people are, but it's important to know your individual levels, before you can decide what actions you need to take for better health.

If you are not getting out in the sun almost daily and not eating appropriate vitamin D-rich foods or taking supplements, you are at high risk for a deficiency and the myriad diseases that can result.

The best way to know if you are deficient is to have a yearly (or better, twice yearly) measurement of 25-hydroxyvitamin D as part of your annual physical examination.

Many people have their cholesterol checked every year, although the evidence that cholesterol levels increase heart attack risk is controversial. Optimal levels of vitamin D are far more important to overall health than low cholesterol, but hardly anyone routinely checks their levels of the sunshine vitamin.

Take Action: Get Your Levels Tested

At the end of each chapter in this book, you get actionable advice, often with steps you can take to increase your health. These are things you can actually do… not just read about.

In the first chapter, you began paying more attention to the sun's cycles, and you to began taking a morning walk when the sun's rays are at their gentlest. In the second chapter, you discovered how important it is to check facts rather than buy into the misleading claims of the "sun police."

Your next step toward better health is to get your vitamin D levels tested. If you haven't been to your doctor in the last year make an appointment today. If you have an appointment scheduled, write a note to yourself reminding you to request a vitamin D test.

The test you should ask for is a 25-hydroxyvitamin D test. This test measures levels of calcidiol in your blood and is the only test you should use to determine vitamin D deficiency. There is a second test that measures calcitriol, but the 25(OH)D test is a much better marker for overall health.

Optimal 25-hydroxyvitamin D values are:	Normal 25-hydroxyvitamin D lab values are:
50-60 ng/ml or 125-160 nmol/l	8-60 ng/ml 20-150 nmol/l

If you're concerned your doctor won't support you in your decision to test your vitamin D levels, you can arrange to have the test done without a doctor's appointment. You can visit DirectLabs.com to learn more. One advantage to a home test is that you can analyze your results. Doctors rarely use optimum levels as their guide. Instead they look at anything within the normal range as fine, even though levels in the low range of normal can substantially increase your risk of disease and health complications.

Also remember, when looking at your results that you may see some seasonal variations. In other words, your levels will likely be lower in the winter than in the summer. It's best to measure your levels twice a year, once at the end of winter when your levels are lowest, and once at the end of summer when your levels are highest. At the very least, you should get an annual measurement.

> ## What Kind of Test Should I Ask My Doctor for?
>
> There are several companies that make 25(OH)D tests. The gold standard is from the company DiaSorin. They are so reputable that the largest commercial lab in the U.S., Quest Diagnostics, trusts only DiaSorin 25(OH)D tests.

Don't wait. Arrange today, to have your vitamin D levels checked. This one hormone can dramatically reduce your chances of developing a chronic disease… and if your levels are low, it's easy to fix.

Let's look at exactly how in the next chapter.

(Endnotes)

1 Peterlik M, Cross HS. (2005). <u>Vitamin D and calcium deficits predispose for multiple chronic diseases.</u> *Eur J Clin Invest.* 35(5):290-304.

2 Peterlik M, Cross HS. (2005). <u>Vitamin D and calcium deficits predispose for multiple chronic diseases.</u> *Eur J Clin Invest.* 35(5):290-304.

3 Zittermann A. (2003). Vitamin D in preventive medicine: are we ignoring the evidence? *Br J Nutr.* 89(5):552-72.

4 Cannell, J. (2006). The secret of Vitamin D production. The Vitamin D Council. http://www.mercola.com/2005/feb/2/vitamin_d_production.htm

Reclaim Your Most Ancient Hormone

CHAPTER FOUR

Diagnose Your Vitamin D Deficiency

"The government has ignored this because it is a political body. The medical community ignores it because they don't have the time nor inclination to read the studies. The drug companies ignore it for economic reasons."

– Dr. John Cannell, MD, The Vitamin D Council

Only in the last decade have we had blood test that could measure levels of vitamin D. It wasn't until then that the negative impact of the ubiquitous 'avoid sunlight' message became fully apparent.

These blood tests turned up widespread deficiencies in people across the country. And, a vitamin D deficiency is a serious condition that you should take measures to guard against.

The best understood consequences of vitamin D deficiency involve the bones. In children, vitamin D deficiency can lead to rickets, a condition where bones don't harden properly. Rickets can result in bowed legs and other deformities.

Reversing Osteoporosis with Sunlight

Sunlight can actually reverse osteoporosis. A lot of senior citizens are taking calcium supplements but not getting enough sunlight, so the calcium is passing right through their bodies. As a result, they are losing bone mineral density.

However, by adding vitamin D through sunlight senior citizens can start assimilating calcium and rebuild their bones.

The same condition in adults is called osteomalacia. The symptoms are weakness, fatigue and chronic pain, especially in the back, hips, chest and ribs. Osteoporosis (brittle bones) is also a sign of vitamin D deficiency.

The Conditions Clearly Associated
Vitamin D Deficiency

- Adrenal insufficiency
- Alzheimer's and Parkinson's
- Allergies
- Autism
- Autoimmune disorders including multiple sclerosis and rheumatoid arthritis
- Blood clotting abnormalities
- Bone and muscle pain
- Cancers of the colon, breast, skin and prostate (and 14 other cancers, including melanoma!)
- Deafness
- Depression, schizophrenia and seasonal affective disorder (SAD)
- Diabetes, Type I and II
- Fibromyalgia and chronic fatigue
- Gluten and lectin intolerance
- Grave's disease
- Heart disease and hypertension
- Infertility, sexual dysfunction
- Immune suppression
- Increased infection
- Insomnia
- Kidney disease
- Liver disease
- Learning and behavior disorders
- Lupus erythematosis
- Metabolic Syndrome, decreased glucose tolerance and insulin sensitivity
- Misaligned teeth, periodontal disease and cavities
- Muscular sclerosis
- Myopia
- Obesity
- Osteoporosis, osteomalacia, Rickets
- PMS
- Psoriasis
- Rheumatoid arthritis
- Thyroid dysfunction
- Vision loss

But few knew until recently that these bone diseases are just the beginning of a long list of chronic diseases and major health complications linked to low vitamin D levels. Below you'll see just a partial list of the hundreds of conditions associated with vitamin D defiency.

How to Know if You Have Vitamin D Deficiency?

In the last chapter, you learned how to test your vitamin D levels. Now let's consider how we determine what is normal, optimal, and deficient?

One tool to get an idea of what is "normal" and what is "deficient," is to look at populations living near the equator where we all evolved from. At or near the equator, the average person has vitamin D levels around 50 ng/ml. All evidence suggests that these are in close range to those of past generations who lived and worked in the sun.

We can think of levels of deficiency ranging to optimum levels in graduations:

- Extreme deficiency: 20 ng/ml (high risk of various conditions)
- Clinically deficient: below 32 ng/ml (increased risk of various conditions)
- Borderline deficient: below 35 ng/ml
- Acceptable: 35-45 ng/ml
- Healthy: 45-55 ng/ml or
- Optimal: 55 ng/ml
- Excess: greater than 100 ng/ml
- Intoxication: greater than 150 ng/ml

People do suffer from extreme deficiency these days. And it's very common to find people with a clinical or borderline deficiency. Ideally, you want to maintain a healthy year-round level of around 50 ng/ml.

Widespread Vitamin D Deficiency Has Reached Epidemic Levels

Vitamin D deficiency is truly reaching a crisis. In fact, one recent study suggests that half of Europeans are deficient and that more than 1 billion people worldwide are deficient in this vital nutrient.

- New studies document dangerously low levels in American children. In fact rickets, a disease that was thought to be wiped out, is making a comeback.

- Breastfed infants will be deficient if their mothers are (and most mothers are).

- Vitamin D deficient infants and children may be imprinted for life with an increased risk of type 1 diabetes, 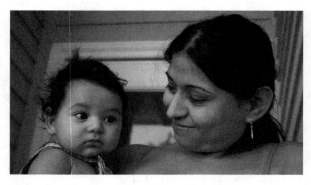 schizophrenia, multiple sclerosis, rheumatoid arthritis, osteoporosis and a number of common cancers.

- Another study conducted in Boston found a high degree of deficiency in white (30%), Hispanic (42%) and black (84%)

elderly people at the end of August when levels should be at their peak.[1]

- In minorities, the elderly, the chronically ill and pregnant women, the problem is nearly universal.

- Eighty-nine percent of the population is deficient in calcium, vitamin D, or both.[2]

Determining if You Are at Risk

If you get very little sunlight on exposed skin and don't supplement your diet with vitamin D, you probably have a deficiency. This puts you at greater risk for disease. Your overall risk depends on a number of factors including where you live, your age, your skin type, your weight and your lifestyle.

Risk Factors:

Where You Live – In mid to higher latitudes, UV-B radiation is limited during the fall, winter and spring months. In his book, the *UV Advantage*, Dr. Holick divides the earth into four climactic regions. Any area north of 35° latitude (or south of the corresponding latitude in the southern hemisphere) will not receive enough UV radiation to trigger adequate vitamin D production for approximately six months out of the year. For Americans this is anywhere above Atlanta, Georgia.

The atmosphere readily filters UV-B radiation. This means that any time the sun is at a low angle in the sky, your body won't produce much vitamin D. So higher latitudes, early morning and late afternoon sun, and winter months all mean less vitamin D.

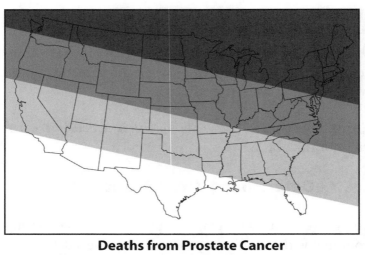

Deaths from Prostate Cancer

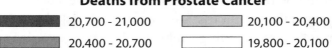

20,700 - 21,000	20,100 - 20,400
20,400 - 20,700	19,800 - 20,100

Your Age – As your skin ages, you need more sun exposure to create vitamin D. For example, expose a 70-year old and a 20-year old to the same amount of sunlight and the 70-year-old will only make about 25% of the vitamin D as the 20-year old. The elderly also have more difficulty metabolizing vitamin D in the liver and kidneys.

Your Skin Type – Dark skin, or skin that doesn't easily sunburn, is a natural adaptation to block ultraviolet rays. This is beneficial if you live outdoors, nearly naked year-round in the tropics, but if you have dark skin mostly covered with clothes, and live indoors in a northern region, you're at a distinct disadvantage when it comes to vitamin D. A person with dark skin requires 10-50 times more sun to produce the same amount of vitamin D as a person with light skin![3]

People with darker skin have a higher risk of a number of diseases because of this. Research shows that people with dark skin:

Diagnose Your Vitamin D Deficiency

- Have higher rates of internal cancer than fair-skinned people living in the exact same areas.[4]
- Are more likely than their fair-skinned counterparts to suffer heart disease and stroke.
- Are four times more likely to die from complications related to high blood pressure than people with light skin.[5]

In fact, in 2002 the U.S. Centers for Disease Control reported that severe vitamin D deficiency is 24 times more common among young black women than it is among young white women. If you have dark skin and live in the northern latitudes, get your vitamin D levels tested and then make a plan to lift your levels accordingly.

Cancer More Prevalent Among African Americans

Cancer rates are still higher among African Americans compared to their Caucasian counterparts, according to a recent statistic released by the American Cancer Society. African Americans die from skin cancer at rates that far exceed Caucasians. Since dark pigmentation blocks vitamin D synthesis in the skin, as many as 75 percent of American Americans are chronically deficient in the anticancer vitamin.

Most forms of cancer are more prevalent in African Americans versus Caucasians on an adjusted scale per 100,000 people, however the few exceptions are cancers of the breast, skin, bladder and also leukemia, the report shows.

Your Weight – Obesity raises your risk of vitamin-D deficiency. There is a biological reason for this. Vitamin D is stored in body fat. And if you are obese, vitamin D can become trapped within body fat making it unavailable to the bloodstream.

Your Lifestyle – If your occupation or lifestyle prevents you from spending at least 15 to 20 minutes in the sunlight an average of three to five days a week, then you're at increased risk for deficiency. Likewise, if you always stay covered up or if you rarely spend time in the sun without sunscreen, you have an increased risk of vitamin D deficiency. **A sunscreen with an SPF of 8 reduces vitamin D production by 95%!**

Diseases and Medications – Certain diseases reduce your body's ability to make vitamin D or to use the vitamin D it has. Pancreatic enzyme deficiency, Crohn's disease, cystic fibrosis, celiac disease, liver disease, hepatic disease, and kidney disease can all interfere with the vitamin D systems in your body. Medicines like phenytoin, phenobarbitol, and rifampin accelerate the breakdown of vitamin D by the liver.

Consider all of these risk factors. If you appear in a high risk group, follow through on the advice at the end of the previous chapter to get your vitamin D levels tested. As you continue to read this book, you'll get a detailed plan to optimize your levels even if you are deficient now.

Begin Optimizing Your Vitamin D Levels Today to Prevent Disease and Boost Health

So, we've looked at what qualifies as a vitamin D deficiency. We've explored the diseases a deficiency can cause or contribute to. And we've looked at what puts you at risk for a vitamin D deficiency in the first place.

But how much vitamin D do you need to get each day to prevent a deficiency?

According to Dr. John Cannell, MD of the Vitamin D Council,

"Adults in the north could take one 5,000 unit capsule a day in late fall, winter, and early spring,

less in the late spring and early fall, and none in the
summer months - depending on your sunning habits.
Children over 50 pounds need 2,000 units each day in
the colder months, while children under 50 pounds
need about 1,000 units per day in the colder months."

In the summer months, getting enough vitamin D shouldn't be a problem. A young adult with fair skin makes 20,000 units of vitamin D in just minutes of sun exposure... provided they aren't covered in sunscreen. This is five times the maximum amount that the Institute of Medicine (IOM) claims is safe to consume, but, of course, your body knows best.

In the winter months, you need to take more specific action to get adequate vitamin D. In one study performed at Creighton University in Omaha, researchers found that adults will use 3,000 to 5,000 units of vitamin D a day, if it is available to your body.[6] These same researchers also concluded that the current recommended daily allowance (RDA) of vitamin D is grossly insufficient.

So let's say, you've identified that you're at risk of vitamin D deficiency. Or you have a blood test and find out you are severely deficient. Perhaps you live in a location

The Government's Inadequate Daily Recommendations:

- 200 IU of vitamin D for infants 0-12 months of age
- 200 IU for males and females 1-50 years of age
- 400 IU for those 50 to 70 years old
- 600 IU for people over the age of 70

where you can't raise your vitamin D level by sunshine alone. How much vitamin D can you take safely in a supplement form? And do you need to be concerned about taking too much vitamin D?

Well, let's find out…

Our Government Missed the Boat about How Much You Need

In 1997, the Food and Nutrition Board of the Institute of Medicine set the recommended daily allowance for vitamin D (see sidebar). The amount of vitamin D the government recommends is woefully short of the amount you need.

From many different pieces of research and from the reality of widespread deficiencies, we now know *the government levels simply aren't adequate.* Without adequate sunlight, these supplemental levels will prevent only the most severe deficiencies.

These levels might provide minimum protection against the development of rickets in children, but they do not come close to the amount of vitamin D needed to maintain optimal health.[7]

Look at the facts:

1. **How much vitamin D your body makes when exposed to sunlight** – During the summer months, if you expose most of your body to direct sunlight until your skin turns very slightly pink, your body will produce approximately 20,000 units of vitamin D. This is 100 times greater than the recommended daily allowance (RDA). It's the equivalent of taking 50 multi-vitamins or drinking 200 glasses of milk!

2. **The amount your body uses on a daily basis** – In 2003, the study at Creighton University found that a healthy young adult body will utilize between 3,000 and 5,000 units of vitamin D[8] (if it is available in the body).

In other words the amount the body actually uses on a daily basis is 20 times more than the government says you need!

After a review of numerous studies, it appears that 4,000 IU of vitamin D per day, from all sources, is about optimal. If you get some (but not a lot) of sun exposure, then you probably only need to consume about 2,000 IU per day from food and supplements. Of course, your best option is to spend 20 minutes to an hour in the sun as often as possible. If you supplement with vitamin D, it is a good idea to get your blood tested twice a year, and take enough to maintain 50 ng/ml year round.

If you are severely vitamin D deficient, or battling an illness, substantially more vitamin D may be required for a period of time. Many patients have taken doses of 50,000 IU for a week or more, and then scaled back to a maintenance dose of 5,000 IU per day. In any case, supplementing with anything over 5,000 IU per day should only be done under a doctor's supervision and only if you intend to test your blood levels intermittently to avoid excess.

Can Too Much Vitamin D Be Toxic?

"Worrying about vitamin D toxicity is like worrying about drowning when you are dying of thirst."

– Dr. Reinhold Veith

Why do our government guidelines propose such a low amount of vitamin D? We read much about the fear of toxicity but little about the consequences of our widespread deficiency. There has been such paranoia about vitamin D toxicity, that physicians are on record warning that just a few too many supplemental doses could prove toxic.

Because this can be a source of confusion, let's clear up the facts about vitamin D toxicity.

Should You Fear Vitamin D Toxicity?

Too much vitamin D can become toxic. Vitamin D toxicity develops over a period of time and usually requires months of excessive doses to manifest.

Vitamin D toxicity can cause:

- Calcium deposits in soft tissues
- Irreversible kidney damage
- Calcium loss from bone
- Premature heart attack and hardening of the arteries
- Vomiting
- Anorexia
- Headaches

Early symptoms include:

- Nausea
- Vomiting
- Decreased appetite
- Constipation
- Weakness
- Weight loss
- Confused mental state
- Heart arrhythmia

So, yes, vitamin D toxicity is very serious. But the government's stance that 2,000 units of vitamin D a day is toxic just isn't so.

In 1999 Dr. Reinhold Vieth of the University of Toronto established that the fear over vitamin D toxicity among conventional doctors is unwarranted. He found no evidence within scientific literature that even 10,000 units of vitamin D per day is toxic. In all the published literature concerning vitamin D toxicology, Vieth could not find anything to indicate toxicity occurring at doses lower than 20,000 units a day.[9]

Vieth's research indicates that toxicity only begins to develop with long-term consumption of approximately 40,000 units of vitamin D per day.[10] He even challenged medical researchers around the world to present a single case of vitamin D toxicity in adults from ingestion of up to 40,000 IU a day. No one has come forward with such a case. If anything, all of the research since has only confirmed Vieth's findings.

The government says: Anything over 2,000 units of vitamin D a day may be toxic.

Common sense says: How could 2,000 units a day be toxic if your body can naturally make 10 times that amount[11] simply by venturing into the sunlight for half an hour or so?

Although numerous studies already existed to show that it would take a significant daily dose of vitamin D consumed over a long period to induce toxicity, the IOM chose to ignore the evidence in favor of a single study. By every indication, this study was greatly flawed.

In this particular study[12] conducted in India in 1984, a Dr. Narang and his colleagues determined that 3,800 units per day of vitamin D, administered over a period of time became toxic. The only problem was that Dr. Narang never measured the amount of vitamin D he gave his subjects! He simply relied on the label to tell him. It now appears that Dr. Narang had given his subjects about 100 times the amount he thought he did.

Unfortunately, the IOM's reliance on this single study resulted in a prevailing misunderstanding of how much vitamin D the body needs.

Who Should Avoid Vitamin D

There are certain conditions, in which people shouldn't take Vitamin D. People with primary hyperparathyroidism, sarcoidosis, granulomatous disease, or other conditions that cause high blood calcium can easily suffer vitamin D toxicity.

If you suffer from any disease associated with an alteration of the vitamin D endocrine system, such as sarcoidosis, do not take any D from any source and avoid sunlight. Persons with any type of liver or kidney disease should consider vitamin D supplementation only if working with a knowledgeable physician.

Otherwise, you need vitamin D daily not monthly or weekly. Your body does best with a steady supply. If you live down south, you can go in the sun for a few minutes every day. If you live up north you can sun in the warmer months and use a sunlamp or take real vitamin D (cholecalciferol) in the winter.

Let's look at the best ways to boost your vitamin D levels.

Sunlight is Your Best Source

Obviously, by far the safest and most effective way to get vitamin D is from the sun. With the sun, you don't have to worry about toxicity because it's impossible to get too much vitamin D. Not a single case has ever been found of vitamin D toxicity from sunlight.

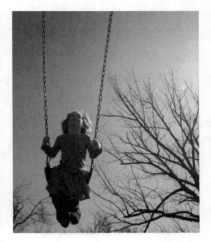

If you live far from the equator, or have other risk factors for a vitamin D deficiency, then you need other sources of vitamin D that are safe and effective.

If you consistently get moderate sun exposure, you shouldn't have to worry about your vitamin D levels. Unfortunately, most of us work indoors or live in places where there's not enough UV-B radiation to produce the amount of vitamin D our bodies need. This is true for more than half of the United States and all of Europe for much of the year (excluding summer).

The Best Ways to Get More Vitamin D in Winter

When you can't get enough vitamin D from the sun, dietary supplements are your next best bet. Most people should supplement in the late fall, winter, and early spring. You should also consider supplementing year round if you have darkly pigmented skin, are over 65, if you're overweight, or if you just can't bring yourself to go into the sun without sunscreen.

You can start by adding a good quality multivitamin to your daily routine. But most multivitamins are only a start. The average multi contains 400 international units of vitamin D. This is only 10 to 20 percent of what you need.

Beyond a multi-vitamin, you can take a dedicated vitamin D supplement. Just make sure that it contains only the natural form of vitamin D3. This will be listed as cholecalciferol on the label.

Two companies that make vitamin D supplements we recommend are Carlson's and Bio-Tech Pharmacal. Carlson's brand is carried in many health food stores and they have a product that contains 2,000 IU in one small gel cap. Their website is www.carlsonlabs.com. Bio-Tech Pharma is a federally licensed, FDA approved manufacturer and they produce pharmacological doses of vitamin D in 1,000, 5,000 and 50,000 IU strengths. Their website is www.bio-tech-pharm.com.

Will Using a Tanning Bed Raise My Levels of Vitamin D?

Some forms of artificial light can produce vitamin D in the skin. The problem is that you don't really know what you are being exposed to – including electromagnetic radiation and excess UV-A rays.

Some artificial sun lamps produce significant amounts of UVB and have been shown to raise calcidiol levels into the healthful range. A company called Sperti, makes a lamp that can raise vitamin D levels and has very low levels of UVA rays. Just like the sun, these lamps can't raise vitamin D to toxic levels, but you can overdo your skin exposure and become burned. You'll learn more about different kinds of artificial light in a later chapter.

Please remember that you should never take more than 5,000 IU of vitamin D on a regular basis without consulting a physician and having your blood levels tested. You want to measure your vitamin D levels periodically to make sure that you're succeeding in bringing your levels into a healthy range... and to make sure you're not overdoing it.

Easy-to-Find Food Sources of Vitamin D

You can also get vitamin D from food sources.

Cod liver oil is the most concentrated natural food source of vitamin D. One tablespoon contains about 1,200 to 1,400 IU.

Cod liver oil also offers several other health benefits. It's a rich source of vitamin A.[13] It contains the powerful anti-oxidant co-enzyme Q10 and it is one of the very best sources of beneficial omega-3 essential fatty acids. These cancer and inflammation fighting nutrients are hard to get in sufficient amounts in the modern diet.

Should I be Concerned about Mercury and PCB's if I Take Cod Liver Oil?

Since mercury is water soluble, it may be present in the flesh of fish but it is not present in its oil. Beyond that, all cod liver oils in the US must be approved by the Association of Analytical Communities (AOAC) as free of detectable levels of 32 contaminants before they are imported into this country.

Taking fish oils isn't the same as taking cod liver oil. Although fish oil has omega-3 essential fatty acids it doesn't contain vitamins A and D. What's more, cod liver oil has far more omega-3 fatty acids than your average fish oil. One tablespoon of regular cod liver oil or one-half tablespoon of high-vitamin cod liver oil provides the equivalent of omega-3 fatty acids found in twelve 1,000 mg fish oil capsules!

Vitamin A

Vitamin A is not generally found in foods, but can be found in foods from animals. Plants contain carotenoids (ie., beta-carotene). Yellow and orange vegetables contain significant quantities of carotenoids.

Green vegetables also contain caretenoids, though the pigment is masked by the green pigment of chlorophyll.

A number of good food sources of vitamin A are listed in the table below:

Food	Vitamin A (IU)*
Liver, Beef, cooked, 3 oz	30,325
Raw Carrot, 7-8 in. long	20,250
Carrots, boiled, ½ cup	19,150
Liver, Chicken, cooked, 3 oz	13,920
Sweet Potatoes, baked, 1 medium	8,910
Mango, uncooked	8,050
Green Leafy Vegetables, cooked ½ cup	7,870
Spinach, boiled, ½ cup	7,370
Cantaloupe, raw, ½ of melon	6,800
Kale, boiled, ½ cup	4,810
Pumpkin, ½ cup cooked	3,840
Squash, winter, boiled, ½ cup	3,500
Apricots, 2-3 medium	2,700
Red Pepper, sweet, raw ½ cup sliced	2,620
Watermelon, 1/16 of 10 x 16" melon	2,530
Broccoli, cooked, 2/3 cup or 1 large stalk	2,500
Nectarines, 3 medium	1,650

Diagnose Your Vitamin D Deficiency

Egg Substitute, fortified, ¼ cup	1,355
Peaches, yellow, 1 medium or large	1,330
Instant Oatmeal, fortified, 1 packet	1,050
Tomatoes, 1 medium	1,350
Cherries, 15 large	1,000
Lettuce, green leaf, 2 large or 5 small leaves	950
Asparagus, green 6 stalks, canned	900
Prunes, dried, 4 medium, cooked	510
Fat Free Milk, Vitamin A fortified, 1 cup	500
Cheese Pizza, 1/8 of a 12" pie	380
Milk, whole, 3.25% fat, 1 cup	305
Cheddar Cheese, 1 oz	300
Whole Egg, 1 medium	280

What You Need to Know to
Supplement with Cod Liver Oil

1. **If you live in a tropical climate, work in the sun, or sun-bathe frequently you may not need additional Vitamin D from cod liver oil.** If you already get enough vitamin D from the sun, you can get your omega-3's from fish oil, fatty fish and grass-fed red meat instead.

2. **If you don't get much sun exposure or use sunscreen, you can take cod liver oil year round.** Usually one or two tablespoons of cod liver oil daily with a meal is all you need to maintain healthy levels of vitamin D. Be careful not to combine cod liver oil with other potent sources of vitamin D unless you are actively monitoring your vitamin D blood levels.

3. **Cod liver oil is also rich in vitamin A.** This essential antioxidant vitamin is in its natural form in cod liver oil so there's no concern of toxicity if you don't overdo it.

If you buy cod liver that is not processed into capsules, it has some unique storage requirements. You should only buy cod liver oil in small dark bottles that protect the nutrients inside the oil from spoiling. It should be stored in the refrigerator. And you can further protect the contents by using a wine saver to pull air from the bottle.

Contrary to what many people believe, fresh cod liver oil should not have a foul "fishy" odor or taste. If it does, throw it out... it's beginning to go rancid.

Can You Recommend a High Quality Cod Liver Oil?

Dr. Sears provides an exceptionally high quality cod liver oil harvested from the clean arctic waters of Norway. It has no bad taste or smell. They regularly test the oil using AOAC international protocols by an independent, FDA registered laboratory. It is consistently free of detectable levels of mercury, cadmium, lead, PCB's and other contaminants. You can find it at: www.primalforce.net.

Other Natural Food Sources of Vitamin D

Your body needs cholecalciferol, or vitamin D3. This is the compound your skin makes naturally when exposed to sunlight. The vitamin D in fortified foods such as milk and some supplements often isn't the same as the naturally occurring vitamin D, cholecalciferol.

There are few foods that contain cholecalciferol, and even those that do, contain small amounts. Below is a table of foods that contain natural vitamin D.

Diagnose Your Vitamin D Deficiency

Selected Food Sources of Naturally Occurring Vitamin D[14]		
Food Source	**Amount**	**Vitamin D**
Cod Liver Oil	1 tablespoon	1360 IU
Salmon (cooked)	3.5 ounces	360 IU
Sardines (canned)	3.5 ounces	270 IU
Tuna (canned)	3 ounces	200 IU
Egg (yolk)	1 egg	25 IU
Beef Liver (cooked)	3.5 ounces	15 IU
Swiss Cheese	1 ounce	12 IU

If you're deficient in vitamin D, the first thing you should do is to start consuming more of these foods. Two of the best sources are Alaskan wild salmon and sardines. These fish not only supply a decent amount of vitamin D and omega-3s, they're also free of mercury.

Why You Should Avoid Vitamin D Fortified Foods

What about fortified foods? I'm sure you've heard that fortified milk is a good source of vitamin D. Unfortunately, that's not usually the case. Often fortified foods contain a different form of vitamin D called ergocalciferol or vitamin D2. Now, if you're deficient, any form of vitamin D is preferable to the higher risk of cancer, heart disease and other chronic health problems. Still, the natural form is far superior to the manufactured form.

1. **The manufactured version isn't as potent and doesn't last as long in your body.** The vitamin D found in milk, most fortified foods and even some vitamins is the synthetic version of vitamin D known as ergocalciferol. This man-made version is not nearly as potent, and it doesn't last as long in the body. Research shows the natural form of vitamin D is nearly twice as effective at raising circulating vitamin D levels than the synthetic version.[15]

2. **Synthetic vitamin D is linked to health problems.** Synthetic vitamin D is now added to almost all milk, even baby foods, cereal, pasta, and flour. Already a number of prominent researchers have raised questions about the safety of long term use of synthetic vitamin D.[16] In Dr. Zane Kime's book *Sunlight*, published in 1980, he references a number of studies that link synthetic vitamin D to irritation of the lining of blood vessels.

3. **It's much easier to overdose synthetic vitamin D.** Research shows synthetic vitamin D becomes toxic in the body at far lower levels than natural vitamin D. Some studies also suggest that milk can amplify the effect of synthetic vitamin D. In an experiment involving school children, the effects produced by 90 units of synthetic vitamin D were greater than the effects of ten times that, 900 units of natural vitamin D in the form of cod liver oil.[17]

4. **You can never be sure your body's getting enough.** When Dr. Michael Holick and his colleagues at the Boston University School of Medicine tested samples of milk, they found 8 out of 10 samples contained either 20% less or 20% more vitamin D than the amount the label advertised. And some of the milk tested contained no vitamin D at all![18]

Vitamin D fortified foods are a gamble. As you can see, you don't want to rely on them solely to ensure healthy levels of vitamin D. If you insist on staying out of the sun and refuse to get regular, moderate exposure, it's essential to supplement. However, before supplementing with vitamin D, it's wise to have your levels tested.

The Most Neglected Modern Hormone Deficiency

If vitamin D deficiency is so widespread and so clearly implicated in a variety of different life threatening health problems, why don't most doctors know about it?

While some of the best scientists are doctors, very few doctors are scientists. Doctors don't spend their time in a lab, they spend their time treating patients. Few of them have extra time to keep up with the latest scientific discoveries in all fields of medical study. In fact, new research is so prolific, that trying to follow it all could easily become a full time job in itself.

So doctors skim research to learn what's new. It's unfortunate that researchers with the most money to fund studies and reach out to doctors are the ones backed by drug companies. The sad fact is that unless a drug company has a profit-making reason to promote a new research discovery, they just don't.

When it comes to vitamin D, no matter how beneficial and effective it is, sunlight is free. There's not way to profit from it. Vitamin D itself simply cannot be patented. Most market research will continue to ignore the deficiency unless they develop a patentable analog to natural vitamin D to make it profitable.

Your Step-By-Step Plan for Healthy Levels of Vitamin D

First of all, remember that sunlight is your very best source of vitamin D. It is completely natural, and it will not produce toxicity. (In the next chapters, you'll learn more specifics about safely getting enough sun each day.)

However, for most Americans, even the sun is not an adequate source in the winter. You should still get some sun every day that it is possible in the winter, but you can't count on it to adequately boost your vitamin D.

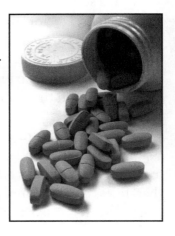

You need dietary sources and possibly a supplement during the late fall, early spring, and winter months. Consider supplementing year round if you are overweight, over the age of 65, have dark skin, or always use sunscreen.

As we've seen, studies show that you can supplement with 3,000 to 5,000 IU of vitamin D a day, and your body will use all of it.

If you take a multi-vitamin, you probably get 400 IU a day. Your body would still use 2,600 to 4,600 more every day if you if it can get it.

One way to get this is to take a daily supplement of just vitamin D. If you do this, here are some guidelines.

1. Aim to take 2,000 IU a day... this leaves room for you to safely get additional vitamin D from other sources like the weak winter sun or from your diet.

2. Take a supplement that contains cholecalciferol (vitamin D3), not ergocalciferol (vitamin D2).

3. One of the best natural sources is cod liver oil. Take one to two tablespoons of cod liver oil a day with food. There is 1200 to 1400 IU of vitamin D in a tablespoon of cod liver oil.

To boost your dietary intake of vitamin D, add Alaskan salmon, sardines, and eggs to your diet. Eggs are a great way to start your day. Despite the cholesterol-phobia that surrounded eggs once upon a time, you can eat one or two eggs each morning without worrying about any negative impact on your health.

Aim to eat salmon and sardines once or twice a week. Wild Alaskan salmon is the cleanest kind of salmon available… it contains little-to-no mercury. It's also versatile, and makes for a tasty dinner. Sardines are readily available in cans. Try topping your salad at lunch with sardines a couple of times each week. Add a spicy vinaigrette, and you've got a tasty meal.

By taking these steps in the wintertime, you can boost your vitamin D to a healthy level year round and dramatically reduce your risks of many chronic diseases.

Remember if you fall into a high-risk category and need to supplement year round, work with your doctor to do this. Your doctor can help you monitor your levels so that you reach your target without overshooting it.

(Endnotes)

1 ImmuneSupport.com. (2006).Vitamin D Deficiency: common cause of many ailments? http://www.immunesupport.com/library/showarticle.cfm/id/6276

2 Eur J Clin Invest. 2005 May;35(5):290-304

3 Holick, MF. (2004). Vitamin D: importance in the prevention of cancers, type 1 diabetes, heart disease, and osteoporosis. *Am J Clin Nutr.* 79(3):362-71.

4 Giovannucci, E. (2005). The epidemiology of vitamin D and cancer incidence and mortality: A review (United States). *Cancer Causes Control.* 16(2):83-95.

5 National Center for Health Statistics: Vital Statistics Report, Final Mortality Statistics, 1969 21:4, US Public Health Service; Rockville, Maryland: 1972.

6 Heany RP, et al. "Human Serum 25-hydroxycholecalciferol response to extended oral dosing with cholecalciferol," *Am J Clin Nutr* 2003; 77(1): 204-10

7 Vieth, R. (1999). Vitamin D supplementation, 25-hydroxyvitamin D concentrations, and safety. *Am.J.Clin.Nutr.* 69:842-56.

8 Heaney, RP et al. (2003). Human serum 25-hydroxycholecalciferol response to extended oral dosing with cholecalciferol. *Am J Clin Nutr.* 77(1):204-10.

9 Vieth, R. (1999). Vitamin D supplementation, 25-hydroxyvitamin D concentrations, and safety. *Am.J.Clin.Nutr.* 69:842-56.

10 Vieth, R, et al. (2001). Efficacy and safety of vitamin D3 intake exceeding the lowest observed adverse effect level. *Am J Clin Nutr.* 73(2):288-94.

11 Holick, MF. (1995). Environmental factors that influence the cutaneous production of vitamin D. *Am J Clin Nutr.* 61(3 Suppl):638S-645S.

12 Narang, NK, Gupta, RC, Jain, MK. (1984). Role of vitamin D in pulmonary tuberculosis. *J Assoc Physicians India.* 32(2):185-8.

13 Cannell, J. (2006). Up to 70 percent of Americans may be deficient in vitamin D- Find out why you don't want to be one of them. The Vitamin D Council. http://www.mercola.com/2003/dec/24/vitamin_d_deficiency.htm

14 National Institutes of Health Office of Dietary Supplements. (2004). Dietary supplement fact sheet: vitamin D. http://ods.od.nih.gov/factsheets/vitamind.asp#h1

15 Trang HM, Cole DE, Rubin LA, Pierratos A, Siu S, Vieth, R. (1998). <u>Evidence that vitamin D3 increases serum 25-hydroxyvitamin D more efficiently than does vitamin D2.</u> *Am J Clin Nutr.* 68(4):854-8.

16 Vieth R, Chan PC, MacFarlane, GD. (2001). <u>Efficacy and safety of vitamin D3 intake exceeding the lowest observed adverse effect level.</u> *Am J Clin Nutr.* 73(2):288-94.

17 Kime, ZR. (1980). *Sunlight.* Penryn, CA: World Health Publications. p. 148-151

18 Holick, MF, Jenkins, M. (2003). *The UV Advantage.* New York, NY: ibooks, Inc. p.149.

CHAPTER FIVE

Beat the Modern Rise of Skin Cancer

"It is clear that squamous cell cancer (SCC) is due almost entirely to sun exposure, that basal cell cancer (BCC) is partly due to sun exposure, and that melanoma is not due to sun exposure."[1]

– Allen J. Christophers

Ask a hundred people *"What's the risk of sun exposure?"* and nearly all of them would mention skin cancer. It's not surprising. For decades, we've been bombarded with messages that the sun causes cancer and should be avoided.

You've heard plenty about the risk of skin cancer from the sun. But did you know that:

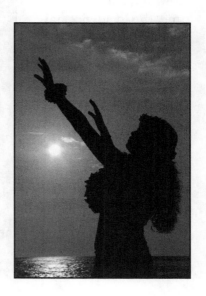

- The most deadly skin cancers, called melanomas, frequently occur on areas of the body not exposed to sunlight?
- There is no link between sun exposure without sunburn and melanoma?
- And, populations with more sun exposure have *less* melanoma?

For example, the very long-lived populations of the Hunzas and the Vilcabambas live at high elevations where the sun is more intense. They spend all day outside, farming. Yet they live to very old ages without getting cancer. If the sun causes skin cancer, how do these people and others like the sun-drenched Polynesians survive?

The answer is that lots of other factors beyond the sun come into play in skin cancer. In this chapter, you'll discover the many factors involved. And, you'll find real strategies to protect your skin from cancer and lower your risks while still enjoying the rays of the sun.

There's More to Skin Cancer than You've Heard

There is no doubt that skin cancer is rampant. It is, by far, the most commonly diagnosed form of cancer and, according to the Centers for Disease Control, well over a million Americans will be diagnosed this year.

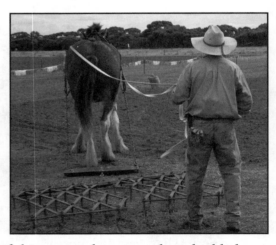

Before the 1930's skin cancer was rare. However, since that time, the incidence has increased drastically. Since 1930, the incidence of melanoma has gone up 1,800 percent. And in just the last 30 years the death rate from melanoma has increased more than four times, while the incidence of all types of skin cancer has more than doubled.

Statistics like these are the first thing that the sunscreen industry and dermatology profession point to as the reason you need sunscreen. But how in the world could these massive increases be "caused" by the sun? The sun certainly hasn't changed in the last 80 years, nor do we receive more sun exposure than we used to.

Consider a few facts:

- At the start of the twentieth century, more than 75% of people across the U.S. worked outdoors.
- Today, in great contrast, only 10% of the U.S. population works outside.
- In the last 30 years our use of sunscreen has dramatically increased.
- Americans are now avoiding the sun, yet skin cancer is the most rapidly increasing form of cancer in the United States.
- Current research suggests that as many as half of Americans who live to 65 will develop some form of skin cancer in their lifetime.[2]

How could sunlight be the only cause of skin cancer, considering that people are getting less sun and more cancer? Logic dictates that the dramatic increase in the incidence of skin cancer cannot solely be explained by exposure to UV-radiation.

To clear the sun of its bad rap, you need to understand skin cancer. There are three very different types:

1. Basal cell carcinoma
2. Squamous cell carcinoma
3. Malignant melanoma.

Let's take a closer look at each…

Basal Cell Carcinoma (BCC) – Basal cell carcinoma is the most common form of skin cancer, accounting for 75 percent of all cases. BCC is characterized by a raised translucent outgrowth, often with a smooth, pearly appearance. These growths sometimes crust and bleed. Some people describe their BCC as a sore that won't heal.

BCC usually develops on parts of the body most frequently exposed to the sun such as the face and hands, but it can appear anywhere. In one large study, researchers from Harvard concluded that increased risk of basal cell carcinoma comes from "blistering sunburn" and is proportional to lifetime sunburn accumulation.[3]

BCC does not spread, but if untreated it can burrow deep into the underlying tissues and cause serious damage. If BCC occurs near the eyes, nose, or ears and spreads into surrounding tissues, it can damage these delicate areas. While BCC is the most prevalent form of skin cancer, it is easily treatable and rarely fatal.

Squamous Cell Carcinoma (SCC) – Squamous Cell Carcinoma is the next most common skin cancer, accounting for about 20 percent of all skin cancers. SCC normally appears as a firm pink or red bump that may become scaly and ulcerated in the center.

These growths may appear anywhere on the body, but like basal cell carcinomas, they most often show up on exposed areas. Squamous cell skin cancer primarily affects people who sunburn easily and tan poorly. This form of skin cancer is more dangerous than basal cell because it can spread to other parts of the body. However, like BCC it is also easily treatable and rarely fatal.

SCC is clearly associated with cumulative sun exposure and usually develops in old age. This type of skin cancer is also associated with intermittent sunburns and people with fair skin have the highest risk of developing SCC.

These two most common forms of skin cancer are relatively benign when compared with other cancers. Removing the lesions sometimes requires delicate surgery and can cause scarring, but they are rarely life threatening.

Beat the Modern Rise of Skin Cancer

The National Institute of Health estimates there are approximately 600,000 cases of BCC and SCC combined in the United States each year. Yet deaths from these two skin cancers only amount to 1,500 Americans a year. And, these are usually cases where detection and treatment was delayed.

Malignant Melanoma – Melanoma is rarer than the other forms of skin cancer, accounting for only 5 percent of cases. It is also much more serious. It can quickly spread throughout the body, and once it begins to spread it is very difficult to beat.

As opposed to the more superficial forms of skin cancer, melanoma originates in the deeper layers of skin tissue, in cells called melanocytes. Melanocytes are the cells that produce the pigment melanin, which colors our skin. Most often, it shows up first in new or pre-existing moles, which are a concentration of melanocytes.

While melanoma can be deadly, it is also highly treatable if you catch it early. This makes it important to know the early signs of melanoma.

Know How the 3 Types of Skin Cancer Compare.[4]			
Skin cancer	**Percentage**	**Prognosis**	**Connection to sunlight**
Basal Cell Carcinoma	75 percent of all skin cancers	Easily treatable and rarely fatal.	Usually appears on the areas exposed to sunlight, and is connected to blistering sunburns.

Squamous Cell Carcinoma	20 percent of all skin cancers	Easily treatable and rarely fatal.	Partly due to sun exposure with a definitive connection to sunburn.
Malignant Melanoma	5 percent of all skin cancers	Accounts for 75 percent of all skin cancer deaths.	Usually on skin not exposed to sun. There is no connection between melanoma and moderate sun exposure.

You should note that there is no link between moderate, sensible sun exposure without burning and skin cancer in any of its forms. So be smart about your sun exposure. You should never allow your skin to burn. But by no means should you avoid the sun

Determine Your Skin Cancer Risk

There is no doubt that sunburn causes damage to the DNA and can lead to cancer. However an expanding body of science now tells us that the **sun is only a co-factor** – one of many contributing factors – and even then, it is only when you overdo your sun exposure that it plays a role.

The *National Library of Medicine* lists hundreds of peer-reviewed medical studies related to the development of skin cancer. Among these studies many causes and contributing factors have been identified. In addition to repeated sunburns, skin cancer risk factors include diet, smoking, excessive alcohol consumption, stress, immune suppression, genetics, skin type, and many more. Now let's consider these factors.

Beat the Modern Rise of Skin Cancer

1) Sunburn – When researchers study skin cancer in animals, they expose them to powerful UV rays over short periods of time, the equivalent of an intense sunburn. Research shows that exposure to the same amount of light over an extended period of time doesn't have the same affect… it doesn't increase skin cancer risks.

Consistent moderate exposure is very, <u>very</u> unlikely to cause cancer. Only repeated sunburns pose a real risk. Whether early sunburns contribute to melanoma later in life is in debate. Some studies point to childhood sunburns[5][6] while other researchers say there's no evidence that childhood sun exposure induces melanoma late in life.[7]

2) Diet and Nutrition – If you eat too many polyunsaturated fats (primarily from vegetable oils) and don't consume enough antioxidants, you increase your risk for developing all of the types of skin cancer. We will have much more to say on this later in this chapter.

3) Smoking – Smoking increases your risk of skin cancer and the more you smoke, the higher the risk. A study conducted in the Netherlands found that current smokers were 3.3 times more likely to develop squamous cell carcinoma. They also found a clear link between the number of cigarettes smoked daily and the chances of developing the disease.[8] Another study showed the risk of skin cancer for current smokers is 50% higher than for those who never smoke.[9]

4) Family History – If you have close relatives with skin cancer, you're more likely to develop the disease. If you've previously had a cancerous lesion, you are also at higher risks of subsequent lesions. But even with a genetic disposition or history of skin cancer, it isn't inevitable that you'll get it. Reduce your other risk factors and your risk will also decline.

5) Skin type – If you have a light complexion and sunburn easily, you have a higher risk of all forms of skin cancer. The sun is still highly important for your health, but you produce vitamin D very rapidly and therefore need only a few minutes in the sun to give your body the vitamin D it needs.

6) Immunity – You have a greater skin cancer risk if your immune system is compromised due to illness or chronically poor nutrition. For example, organ transplant patients whose immune systems are purposely suppressed, experience a much higher risk of skin cancer.[10]

7) Chemical exposure and chlorine – A number of studies show that occupational and environmental exposure to a variety of chemicals and some pharmaceutical drugs increase the risk of the less severe skin cancers. Frequent swimming in chlorinated pools and exposure to chlorination byproducts[11] is also believed to increase melanoma risk.[12]

In a later chapter, we'll explore the link between the toxic chemicals in most sunscreens and the risk of skin cancer.

8) A large number of atypical moles – If you have a high number of moles, large moles, or moles that are irregularly shaped, you have a higher risk of skin cancer.

9) Over consumption of alcohol – Heavy alcohol consumption may increase your risk of melanoma. In one study, people that drink an average of two or more drinks a day showed a higher risk of melanoma.[13]

10) Vitamin D deficiency – If you're deficient in vitamin D, your risk for melanoma rises. Numerous research papers show that breakdown products or derivatives of active vitamin D can actually suppress the growth and spread of malignant melanoma cells.

Beat the Modern Rise of Skin Cancer

11) Obesity – If you are overweight and sedentary, you are at higher risk of melanoma.[14] On the other hand, *increasing your daily amount of exercise can reduce your risk.*

Many of the risk factors for skin cancer are under your control and there are many ways to decrease your risk. You can improve your diet. You can increase your exercise. You can limit your alcohol intake. You can quit smoking. And you can get responsible – not excessive – sun exposure.

And while using sunscreen can protect you from sunburn, don't expect it to provide protection against skin cancer. After a review of the medical literature, Dr Robin Marks, a dermatologist and professor at the University of Melborne said, "There is no substantial evidence that sunscreen protects against any of the three forms of skin cancer. Relying on synthetic chemicals to prevent cancer is laughable." Another dermatologist, Arthur Rhodes of the University of Pittsburgh told a 1994 meeting of the American Cancer Society that sunscreens "appear weakly effective or ineffective" at preventing cancer.

The Truth about Melanoma and the Sun

The Sun Police lump all skin cancers together. But as you have seen, sun exposure plays a very different role in different types of skin cancers. Most of the studies that link skin cancer to sun exposure are about BCC and SCC. Melanoma, however, is the most feared form of skin cancer and you might be surprised to learn that a suntan is actually protective against this disease.

Dozens of studies, including one review of more than 50 research papers[15] show that people whose occupations keep them indoors have a much higher incidence of melanoma than do those who work outside. For example, office workers have higher rates of malignant melanoma than construction workers, lifeguards or farmers.[16] [17] [18]

Population studies also *clearly* show an inverse relationship between UV exposure and melanoma. For example, rates of melanoma are higher in Minnesota than Arizona, and higher in Norway than the South of France.

Why Do We Use Study Results?

Whenever you are researching some critical aspect of your health, it's important to know where information comes from and what research studies back it up.

Research studies help us:

- Illustrate how diseases develop.
- Identify why diseases occur in some individuals and not others.
- Know what treatments work.

When multiple studies come to similar conclusions, you can have a greater degree of confidence in their findings. The information in this book is backed by over 200 citations to scientific articles and peer reviewed research studies.

Another inconvenient truth that calls the role of sunlight into question is the fact that melanomas frequently occur on areas of the body that are the *least* exposed to sunlight – chronically shaded areas such as the soles of the feet, under the nails, on the delicate tissues inside the nose and mouth or on the genitals. In Japan, 40% of melanomas are on the feet or soles of the feet. [19]

Take a look at what the studies *really* have to say about melanoma:

- **Those working outdoors have the lowest risk of melanoma** – In 1982, the British medical journal *The Lancet* reported on the relationship between skin cancer and sun exposure. The researchers found that those whose main activity was outdoors had the *lowest risk* of developing malignant melanoma.

Beat the Modern Rise of Skin Cancer

Other studies have yielded the same results. An overview of all of the published research reported in the *International Journal of Cancer* revealed that multiple studies show that people with "heavy occupational exposure" to the sun have significantly lower risk of melanoma.[20]

- **High lifetime recreational sun exposure lowers your risk** – Additional studies performed at the British Columbia Cancer Agency confirmed that the higher your lifetime recreational sun exposure, the lower your risk of melanoma.

- **Lifeguards in Australia have the lowest rates of melanoma** – In the February 2005 issue of the *Journal of the National Cancer Institute* a study confirmed that exposure to the sun reduces the risk of skin cancer.[21] Additional studies have shown that lifeguards in Australia have the lowest rates of melanoma.

- **The incidence of malignant melanoma is twice as high in office workers** – In another study published in *Lancet*, researchers at the University of Sydney's Melanoma Clinic found the incidence of malignant melanoma was twice as high in office workers than those whose occupations or life-style kept them in the sun regularly. Those who had the lowest incidence were sunbathers! Another study showed that those who work under fluorescent light double their risk.[22]

- **A tan can actually help prevent melanoma.** Several studies conclude that a deep tan, particularly in childhood and the adolescent years, provides protection against melanoma.[23] [24] [25]

The combination of these studies plainly indicates that those who spend *more* time in the sun (without burning) have *less* risk of melanoma – quite the opposite of what the anti-sun proponents would have you believe. We can only come to two conclusions based on these findings:

1. A suntan and consistent, moderate exposure to sunlight is protective against melanoma, while intermittent, burning exposure increases the risk.

2. Vitamin D, which is highly protective against internal cancers, is also protective against melanoma. In fact, this has even been proven in the lab, where vitamin D was shown to cause melanoma cells to self-destruct.[26] [27]

So, now you know that healthy sun exposure will actually protect you against deadly melanoma. And you know that there are numerous risk factors for skin cancer. But the question remains, *why is the rate of skin cancer skyrocketing?*

Understanding the REAL Causes of Skin Cancer

The truth is that the increase in skin cancer is related to relatively recent changes in the human diet. Science proves that there are some foods – foods that modern populations eat in abundance – which strongly *promote* skin cancer. On the other hand, there are other foods which strongly *prevent* skin cancer that are in short supply in the modern diet.

When foods that promote skin cancer are eaten in excess and nutrients that prevent it are absent, the skin becomes far more vulnerable to sunlight. In other words, we have artificially *raised* our risk factors for skin cancer, while simultaneously *removing* our natural defenses against it.

To understand how to prevent (and reverse) skin cancer, you must understand how it arises in the first place. Ultimately, the *cause* of skin cancer is oxidative stress.

Beat the Modern Rise of Skin Cancer

The Role of Free Radicals in Skin Cancer

Like all healthy cells, skin cells are rich in oxygen. When your skin is exposed to sunlight, the ultraviolet rays strike these oxygen molecules and can cause some of them to lose an electron. The end result is the oxygen free radical.

This "oxidation" is the same chemical reaction that causes metal to rust or an apple slice to turn brown. Many forms of cancer, including skin cancer, can be the result of cell mutations caused by the reactions between free radicals and DNA.

But this is where many researchers stop searching. They simply attribute skin cancer to the free radicals that are formed as a result of sun exposure. But this is not entirely true.

Because oxygen is your primary metabolic fuel, free radicals occur naturally throughout every cell in your body. In fact, free radicals are a necessary part of numerous biological processes. But because they can cause damage if left unchecked, your body has mechanisms to neutralize them and repair their damage.

Free radicals are meant to be controlled by free radical scavengers known as antioxidants. But if antioxidants are in short supply, or if so many free radicals are formed that they overwhelm the antioxidant defense system, then tissue damage, accelerated aging, and eventually, skin cancer can occur.

And, as you will soon see, the standard American diet (which is rapidly becoming the world's diet) is *abundant* in foods that promote free radicals, and it is *deficient* in the foods that provide antioxidant protection against them.

The Dietary Connection to Skin Cancer

There are three primary changes in the modern diet which strongly promote skin cancer:

1. The over-consumption of sugar and refined carbohydrates.

2. A dramatic increase in the consumption of omega-6 fatty acids.

3. A lack of antioxidant rich food.

The process is very simple. The excessive consumption of refined carbohydrates and omega-6 fatty acids strongly promotes the formation of free radicals. These free radicals then multiply and set off a cascade of oxidative stress because there are not enough antioxidants to neutralize them.

The first step to slow the aging of your skin and reduce your risk of skin cancer, is to avoid sugar and refined carbohydrates.

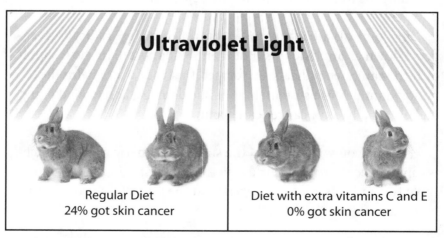

Ultraviolet Light

Regular Diet
24% got skin cancer

Diet with extra vitamins C and E
0% got skin cancer

Diet affects incidence of skin cancer in experimental animals.

Refined Carbohydrates:
The Cancer Connection

There are several reasons that a diet high in sugar and refined carbohydrates increases your risk of cancer. Primarily, it is because these foods dramatically increase inflammation and oxidative stress in the body.

Carbohydrate consumption also stimulates the release of insulin. Cancer cells have six to ten times more insulin receptors than normal cells and it has been said that insulin stimulates the growth of cancer like gas on a fire. Excess sugar in the bloodstream also creates a perfect feeding ground for cancerous cells because glucose is the primary fuel of cancer cells.

Keeping your blood sugar levels low is a critical step towards controlling the ability of cancer to thrive. But there is another risk factor related to skin cancer that is just as important. It has to do with the type of fats you eat.

The Role of Dietary Fat and Skin Cancer

The amount of fat we consume has not changed much over the last hundred years. But the *type* of fat we eat has changed drastically. At the turn of the last century, we ate mostly animal fats, which are primarily saturated and monounsaturated.

But as the technology became available to mass produce oil from seeds and grains, our consumption of polyunsaturated fat began to increase. Then, in the 1950s, in an effort to reduce heart disease, the medical establishment, the processed food industry and the government began an aggressive campaign to steer people away from saturated fats and toward polyunsaturated vegetable oils.

We won't go into the utter fallacy of this idea here, but the end result was that consumption of vegetable oils went through the roof. At the beginning of 1900 there were almost no vegetable oils in our diet. Today, the average American consumes 70 pounds of vegetable fat.

These fats are not a problem when they are contained within the whole food. It is very difficult to consume too much in that form. It is when these fats are extracted and concentrated and then consumed in mass quantities that problems arise. And just look on the nutrition labels, corn oil, soybean oil, peanut oil and many other polyunsaturated fats are in just about every processed food on the grocery store shelf.

You Are What You Eat

We are not designed to eat these fats in the quantities we do. The make-up of fat in the human body is normally about 97 percent monounsaturated and saturated. Only about 3 percent should be polyunsaturated. But the fat in your diet dictates the type of fat in your cells. And if you consume plant oils, your cell membranes will incorporate these fat molecules.

The problem with polyunsaturated fats displacing saturated fats in cell structures is that these fats are highly unstable. This means that they are extremely vulnerable to oxidative stress, especially in the skin, where they are exposed to oxygen and UV light.

The end result is that you will you will sunburn much faster and more intensely[28] and you will also be prone to skin cancer.

Omega-6: The Fat That Promotes Skin Cancer

The polyunsaturated fats in vegetable oils are almost entirely omega-6 fatty acids. When sunlight hits these omega-6 fats, it can easily convert them to cancer-causing molecules.

Among all the foods we eat, omega-6 fatty acids have been shown to be the strongest promoters of skin cancers in both people and animals.[29] In one study performed at the University of Western Ontario, researchers observed the effects of ten different dietary fats ranging from most saturated to least saturated. What they found is that saturated fats produced the least number of cancers, while omega-6 polyunsaturated fats produced the most. Numerous other studies have also shown that polyunsaturated fats stimulate cancer while saturated fat does not[30] and that saturated fats do not break down to form free radicals.[31]

In another study, Dr. Vivienne Reeve, PhD, Head of the Photobiology Research Group at the University of Sydney irradiated a group of mice while feeding different groups of them polyunsaturated and saturated fats. Reeve discovered that the mice that consumed only saturated fat were totally protected from skin cancer, while those in the polyunsaturated fat group quickly developed skin cancers. Later in the study, a soon as the mice in the saturated fat group were given the polyunsaturated fats, skin cancers quickly developed.

But while excessive omega-6 fatty acids promote skin cancer and sunburn (and a host of other health concerns), there is another type of fat that strongly inhibits these things. These are omega-3 fatty acids.

Omega-3 Fats Help to Prevent Skin Cancer

Omega-3 fatty acids are highly beneficial in virtually every aspect of your health. One of their many benefits is that they provide powerful protection against skin aging and skin cancer. This was confirmed in a comprehensive review of many studies published by the National Academy of Sciences in 2001.

One of these studies, performed at the University of Minnesota showed that omega-6 fats promote the risk of skin cancer, while omega-3 fats reduce it.[32] Dr. Lesley Rhodes also explored the ability of omega-3s to protect skin cells. Her research was published in the *Journal of Investigative Dermatology* and it showed that omega-3 fatty acids reduce the inflammation that would normally be induced by excess sun exposure. She also showed that omega-3s significantly reduced DNA damage. This helps to explain why omega-3 fatty acids help to prevent not only sunburn, but skin cancer as well.

In a study published in the journal *Cancer Research* in 2000 researchers showed that the omega-3 fatty acid DHA, inhibited the progression of exponentially growing melanoma cells. This study also noted that omega-6 polyunsaturated fatty acids are known to stimulate skin cancer while omega-3 fatty acids inhibit it:

> *"Epidemiological, experimental, and mechanistic data implicate omega-6 fat as stimulators and long-chain omega-3 fats as inhibitors of the development and progression of a range of human cancers, including melanoma."*

This would help to explain an Australian study which showed a 40% reduction in melanoma for those who frequently eat fish, which is rich in omega-3s.

One of the best things you can do to slow the aging of your skin and prevent skin cancer is to rid your diet of omega-6 ladened plant and seed oils while consuming more protective omega-3 fatty acids. That means you should avoid corn, sunflower, soybean, cottonseed and other vegetable and seed oils, processed foods and conventionally raised meats.

The very best sources of healthy omega-3 fats are cod liver oil and fish oil, which are readily available in supplement form. You should also consume wild Alaskan salmon, grass-fed red meat, sardines, flax seeds and walnuts for their omega-3 content.

Summary of Fats and Skin Cancer

There is no doubt that as a population, we are consuming *less* of the fats that inhibit oxidative stress and *more* of the ones that promote it. These changes have made our bodies predisposed to free radical formation.

And to top it all off, the over consumption of modern processed foods has caused deficiencies in the vitamins, minerals and antioxidants that we need to neutralize the free radicals that are formed. The result is run away oxidative stress and, quite clearly, an epidemic of skin cancer.

Numerous studies have shown that people with a variety of sun-related skin disorders have low levels of antioxidants.

Boost Your Antioxidants for Skin Cancer Protection

In addition to high polyunsaturated fat intake, research clearly shows that low consumption of fruits and vegetables increases your melanoma risk.[33] In one study, researchers at the National Cancer Institute in Bethesda, Md., surveyed 1,000 people, 500 of whom had melanoma. They found that those who

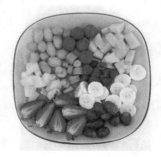

had eaten foods with the most vitamin D and carotenoids, including beta-carotene, cryptoxanthin, lutein and lycopene, had the lowest risk of melanoma.

This should come as no surprise. The role of antioxidants in the protection against many forms of cancer has been clearly established. But it appears that these nutrients are especially protective against skin cancer.

In 1993 the *National Cancer Institute* funded a study of nearly thirty thousand Chinese men and women. The subjects of the study were healthy, but they were part of a population with very high cancer mortality and a low intake of micronutrients. The goal was to determine what effect antioxidant supplements would have on these people.

The intervention very rapidly reduced overall cancer deaths by more than 13 percent. That is a positive result, but not nearly as dramatic as what the researchers discovered about skin cancer. They found that the the incidence of skin cancer fell by a whopping 70 percent.[34]

There are many antioxidants that are highly protective against skin cancer, including vitamins A, C and E, glutathione and alpha lipoic acid (ALA). But it is the carotenoids that provide an extra layer of protection.

Carotenoids: Eat Your Sunscreen

Carotenoids are a family of colorful nutrient molecules that protect plants and animals from excess sunshine. These pigments are literally Mother Nature's sun block.

Carotenoids function in two ways. When you consume carotenoids they are deposited in your skin where they serve to reflect the sun, providing protection against sunburn and skin damage. [35, 36, 37, 38] This helps to prevent cellular damage from occurring in the first place.

But these nutrients are also powerful antioxidants that scavenge for free radicals and repair cells that might become damaged. You could say they reflect and they protect forming a physical barrier and a nutritional barrier against skin damage.

In a German study, volunteers ate 1 tablespoon of tomato paste every day for 10 weeks. When exposed to UV light, the subjects suffered 40 percent less sunburn than volunteers who didn't eat the paste. The researchers concluded that the lycopene (which makes tomatoes red) was responsible.

The leading sources of carotenoids are eggs, spirulina, chlorella, tomatoes, dark green leafy vegetables (kale, collards and spinach) and yellow-orange fruits and vegetables (apricots, cantaloupe, carrots, sweet potatoes, yams, and squash).

Astaxanthin: King of the Carotenoids

The most potent of carotenoids is a red pigment found in salmon, trout, shrimp and lobsters. But the richest natural source of astaxanthin (pronounced asta-ZAN-thin) is microscopic algae. Algae is normally green. But when subjected to UV light, it produces this deep red pigment.

Studies have shown that astaxanthin is hundreds of times more effective at protecting skin from UV damage than other carotenoids! In fact, because of its molecular structure, astaxanthin is one of the most powerful antioxidants ever discovered. This nutrient has been shown to be more than 500 times more effective than vitamin E at preventing fat molecules from forming free radicals.[39, 40] It also boosts your overall antioxidant protection by multiplying the effects of both vitamin E and vitamin C and assisting in their antioxidant activity.[41]

And in addition to its antioxidant activity, this special carotenoid also accumulates under the skin and provides a reflective, protective shield against sunburn and skin damage.

Astaxanthin is also a powerful anti-inflammatory agent and potent immune system builder. It has been shown to enhance and modulate the immune system and also helps the immune system to destroy cancer cells. And not only does it prevent DNA damage, it also increases the activity of the liver enzymes that detoxify carcinogens.[42]

But you don't have to eat algae to get the protection of astaxanthin. It is an inexpensive and readily available dietary supplement. The best selling brand is called BioAstin, made by a company called Cyanotech (www.cyanotech.com). It would be a very wise decision to take this nutrient, especially in the weeks prior to when you might be exposed to more sunshine than normal.

Four Steps to Skin Cancer Protection

So now you know the real reasons for the dramatic increases in the rate of skin cancer. Because of what we eat, we have made ourselves more vulnerable. And because of what we don't eat, we have lost our natural protection.

But these changes in the modern diet are easy to fix. To do so, you must eat a low glycemic diet by reducing the amount of sugar and refined carbohydrates you consume. At the same time, avoid processed foods, conventionally raised meats and vegetable oils.

Eat plenty of healthy fats from wild and naturally raised meats and supplement your diet with fish oil or cod liver oil for the omega-3s. And finally, eat a diet rich in fruits and vegetables and take a few sensible supplements to boost your antioxidant protection.

And don't believe the hype that skin cancer is exclusively caused by the sun. While we're at it, let's put to rest another myth about sun exposure...

Is the Ozone Hole Putting Your Skin at Risk?

Maybe you've heard that we are receiving greater amounts of "dangerous" UV rays than ever before due to the breakdown of the ozone layer. Let's look at the truth behind ozone depletion and any connection it may have to skin cancer.

The ozone is a layer of atmosphere that filters some of the UV radiation from the sun. There is a popular theory that it has become thinner in the last half a century and that holes in the ozone near the planet's poles have been growing.

Some people believe that thinning ozone lets more UVB rays hit the earth, so let's start by looking more closely at the light the earth receives from the sun.

There are three kinds of UV light that reach us from the sun:

- **Ultraviolet-A** (UVA) – These rays make up 90 to 95% of the sunlight that reaches the earth. They have a long wavelength. They penetrate your skin deeply are primarily responsible for the tanning response in your skin.

- **Ultraviolet-B** (UVB) – These rays make up 5 to 10% of the sunlight reaching the earth. UVB rays have a shorter wave-length than UVA rays. They trigger vitamin D synthesis in your skin and are responsible for sunburns.

- **Ultraviolet-C** (UVC) – These rays have the shortest wave-length of all the UV light that comes from the sun. UVC rays are almost completely absorbed by the atmosphere.

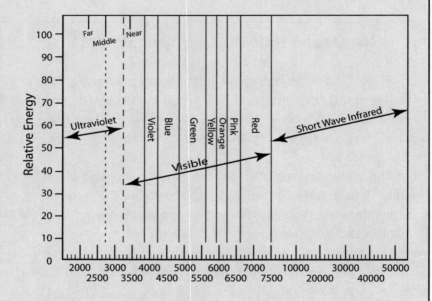

In their book, *The Holes in the Ozone Scare*, authors Rogelio Maduro and Ralf Schauerhammer present a compelling case that the theory of the thinning ozone is false. They believe that much of the fear surrounding increased UV radiation is unwarranted.[43]

3-D imaging tells us that the ozone layer is not uniform in the first place. It is constantly shifting, and there are substantial varia-tions from place to place, from season to season and from year to year. In a paper presented to Congress, Harvard astrophysicist, Sallie Baliunas, said that the natural variability of the ozone layer is "orders of magnitude greater" than the alleged man-made "depletion."

But the fact is that even if the ozone layer *were* thinning, that doesn't explain the increase in skin cancer. Here's why. Even the most vocal proponents of the hole in the ozone theory suggest that ozone depletion has only resulted in an average 10 to 20 percent increase in UV-B radiation at the earth's surface. To give you an idea of what this means, consider the fact that a one percent increase in UVB radiation is the equivalent of moving six miles south of where you are and standing outside. That means a 20 percent increase in solar radiation would be the equivalent of moving 120 miles south. You can actually increase your UV exposure by 100 percent, just by traveling 600 miles south!

That's much more of an effect than ozone depletion could cause, and people do it every day.

Put the Effects of Ozone Depletion into Realistic Terms	
Percentage of increase in UVB Rays	Would be equivalent to:
1%	Moving six miles south
20%	Moving 120 miles south
100%	Moving 600 miles south

You are capable of living in climates with widely varying levels of UVB radiation. For instance:

1. UV-B radiation varies annually by a full 5,000 percent between the Equator and the Poles.

2. Ultraviolet intensity varies 4 to 5 percent every 1,000 feet ascended.

3. Because of these variations, some populations get hundreds of times more solar radiation than others.

4. People all over the world live where ultraviolet light is high, yet they are virtually free from all types of cancer.

While many scientists are concerned about the dangers of the thinning ozone, there are few tests to measure the amount of UV light coming through the holes. The most extensive study to date was conducted by Joseph Scotto in collaboration with the National Cancer Institute. Scotto found that the amount of UVB light reaching ground level stations across the United States had not increased at all.[44]

The Changing Definition of Skin Cancer... and Why it's a Danger to You

How do we define skin cancer? We need to rely on specialists, but this sometimes introduces bias. Remember the old saying that *"To the hammer, everything looks like a nail."*

To illustrate how professional bias can play into our fear, look at this patient's story about her experience at her dermatologist's office:

"Scared by my husband's "precancerous" spot removed from his face, I recently went to the dermatologist for a checkup. After she introduced herself, the first thing she asked me was 'Are you in

*here today because you're worried about skin cancer?'
I acknowledged that I did have a mark on my face I
wanted her to take a glance at.*

*She then started talking about cancer, about how
skin cancer was rampant and how her whole practice
was now built around skin cancer... she admonished
me to wear sunscreen all of the time and that I
needed to be checked yearly.*

*With one more warning about the frequency of skin
cancer, she flew out of the door. A nurse returned with
a bag full of sunscreen samples for me to take with me."*

– from a first-time dermatologist visit, Chicago, Illinois

Remember, melanomas tend to occur on the areas of the body
that are the least exposed to sunlight. Yet these areas aren't the
places dermatologists and other skin professionals focus on when
they consult with patients about fear of skin cancer.

Dermatologists don't worry about internal cancer, diabetes,
seasonal affective disorder (SAD), or any of the other illnesses that
may be prevented by moderate UV exposure. They focus on skin
cancers especially including superficial cancers, which they build a
practice on removing.

In fact, while skin cancers are being diagnosed at more than
double the rate they were in 1986, an article in the New York Times
suggests that perhaps we're "experiencing an epidemic of skin cancer screening" rather than an epidemic of skin cancer.[45]

Dermatologists are now also removing "precancerous patches"
on the skin, further expanding the diagnosis of the disease.

Beware of "Trigger Happy"
Skin Cancer Screening Clinics

In a study published in *The British Medical Journal*, researchers at Dartmouth Medical School discovered that since 1986 skin biopsies have risen by 250 percent.[46] Yet they found no change in the melanoma death rate or in the incidence of melanoma in the advanced stage. Shouldn't more screening decrease the death rate from melanoma?

World-renowned dermatologist, Dr. A. Bernard Ackerman, emeritus director of the Ackerman Academy of Dermatopathology in New York, believes he knows why. In New York Times article, Dr. Ackerman stated that dermatologists are trending toward spending more time removing innocuous moles too readily.

Dr. Ackerman went on to state, "There has been a mania for taking off these moles that are of no consequence. We're talking about billions and billions of dollars being spent, based on hype."[47]

Exposure to Sunlight Aids Cancer Survival

One study designed to show sun exposure causes melanoma produced some surprising results. The study, performed at the University of New Mexico, followed 528 victims of melanoma over a 5-year period. Researchers couldn't find a link between the deadly cancer and sunlight, but they did find that when melanoma victims received moderate sun exposure it doubled their chances of surviving the disease.[48]

How You can Quickly Reduce Your Risk
of Deadly Melanoma

All skin cancers can become serious if left untreated, especially melanoma. All skin cancers, including melanoma can also be successfully removed when caught early. According to the National Cancer Institute, when detected and treated early melanoma is nearly 95 percent curable.[49]

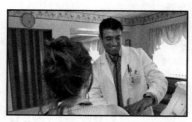

To catch melanoma in an early stage when you can be cured, check your skin regularly. Most melanomas are asymmetrical. They often have an irregular border with scalloped or notched edges. Normal moles generally have a smooth border. Watch for color variation. Melanomas typically have varied shades of brown, tan or black, and may later progress to red, white or blue. Normal moles are usually brown.

Melanomas are often larger than a regular mole. Any mole with a diameter of greater than 6 mm (about the size of a pencil eraser) should be checked, even though melanomas may start smaller than this. Pay attention if you have a mole that changes. Melanomas may change or evolve. If you notice a mole is getting larger, changing shape or color, or that begins to itch or bleed, you should have it looked at by a dermatologist.

Know Your ABC's For Early Melanoma Detection

A. **Asymmetry** – Most melanomas are asymmetrical, where one half of a mole is different from the other.
B. **Border irregularity** – Melanomas often have an irregular border with scalloped or notched edges.
C. **Color variation** – Look for varied shades of brown, tan or black, progressing to red, white or blue within the same lesion.
D. **Diameter** – Pay attention to moles greater than 6 mm (about the size of a pencil eraser).
E. **Evolving** – A mole that is getting larger, that goes from flat to raised, that changes shape or color, or that itches or bleeds is a concern.

Enjoy the Sun Safely and Reduce Your Risk of Skin Cancers and Other Diseases

The main benefit that the sun provides in preventing melanoma and other forms of cancer appears to be its ability to trigger vitamin D production. So the first step is to get responsible sun exposure. But to do that you need to know when the sun will give you the most benefit.

How to Get UV Rays Strong Enough to Make Vitamin D

There are a combination of factors to consider.

1. **Time of day** – The most UV rays are present when the sun is highest at noon.

2. **Time of year** – In northern latitudes, it is virtually impossible to get enough vitamin D from sunlight during the winter months. During the summer, the best hours to maximize vitamin D are during the times of the day you have been told to avoid – from 10 am to 2 pm.

3. **Altitude** – Ultraviolet intensity increases 4% to 5% every 1000 feet ascended. You will get a sunburn faster in the mountains than you will at sea level – the higher up you go, the more UVB rays reach you.

4. **Industry** – Pollution, smog and ozone can block UVB.

5. **Climate** – People who live in cloudy climates with long winters may not get enough vitamin D. If this describes your climate, you will benefit from supplements.

You Don't Need to Burn to Get Your Vitamin D

To maintain healthy skin, you need to be responsible with your sun exposure. Don't allow your skin to burn. Your body produces enough vitamin D for the day in about a quarter of the time it takes for you to begin to sunburn.

Here are some basic guidelines to responsible sun exposure:

1. If you are fair-skinned, 10 to 20 minutes of high summer sun will produce adequate vitamin D levels. If you have skin with a moderate amount of pigmentation, you'll need a bit more... 20 to 40 minutes. Those with the darkest skin may need up to two hours to meet daily vitamin D requirements (or they should take cod liver oil or a vitamin D supplement).

2. Show some skin. When you're working on your vitamin D levels, bare some skin. Show your arms, your shoulders, and your legs when weather and circumstances permit.

3. If you're going to be in the sun longer than what you need for vitamin D, take measures to cover your most sensitive skin – usually your face, shoulders, and the back of your legs.

4. If you're going to spend all day in the sun, after the first hour or so, you'll want to take additional measures to protect the rest of your skin. You'll discover more about choosing safer sunscreens in chapter 15 of this book.

(Endnotes)

1 Christophers, AJ. (1998). Melanoma is Not Caused by Sunlight. *Mutat Res.* 422:113.

2 Schroeder, Sarah. "Benchmarks: Background on Skin Cancer," National Cancer Institute. July 1, 2003.

3 Van Dam, R., *et al., Risk factors for basal cell carcinoma of the skin in men: results from the health professionals follow-up study.* American Journal of Epidemiology, 1999. 50(5): p459-460.

4 "Cloudy Links to Cancer," The LA Times. July 24, 2006

5 Marks, R. (1999). Photoprotection and prevention of melanoma. *Eur J Dermatol.* 9:406.

6 Elwood, JM, Jopson, J. (1997). Melanoma and sun exposure: an overview of published studies. *Int J Cancer.* 73:198.

7 Pfahlberg, A, et al. (2001). Timing of excessive ultraviolet radiation and melanoma: epidemiology does not support the existence of a critical period of high susceptibility to solar ultraviolet radiation- induced melanoma. *Br J Dermatol.* 144(3): p471-5.

8 BBC News. (2000). Smoking 'triples skin cancer risk.' http://news.bbc.co.uk/1/hi/health/1090790.stm

9 Grodstein F, et al. (1995). A prospective study of incident squamous cell carcinoma of the skin in the nurses' health study. *J Natl Cancer Inst.* 87(14):1061-6.

10 Perara GK, et al. "Skin Lesions in Adult Liver Transplant Recipients: a study of 100 Consecutive Patients," *Br J Dermatol* 2006; 154(5): 868-72

11 Bull, RJ, et al. (1985). Evaluation of mutagenic and carcinogenic properties of brominated and chlorinated acetonitriles: by-products of chlorination. *Fundam Appl Toxicol.* 5(6 Pt 1):1065-74.

12 Nelemans, PJ, et al. (1994). Swimming and the risk of cutaneous melanoma. *Melanoma Res.* 4(5):281-6.

13 Freedman DM, et al. "Risk of melanoma in relation to smoking, alcohol intake, and other factors in a large occupational cohort," *Cancer Causes Control* 2003; 14(9): 847-57

14 Grant, W. (2003). Melanoma has a complex etiology that includes UV exposure, skin pigmentation and type, diet, and obesity. BMJ. http://bmj.bmjjournals.com/cgi/eletters/327/7427/1306-b#42706

15 Elwood JM, Jopson J. Melanoma and sun exposure: an overview of published studies. Int J Cancer. 1997 Oct 9;73(2):198-203.

16 Elwood JM, et al. (1985). Cutaneous melanoma in relation to intermittent and constant sun exposure – the western Canada melanoma study. Int J Cancer. 35:427.

17 Elwood, JM. (1992). Melanoma and sun exposure: contrasts between intermittent and chronic exposure. World J Surg.16:157.

18 Garland, FC, et al. (1990). Occupational sunlight exposure and melanoma in the U.S. Navy. Arch Environ Health. 45:261.

19 Groves, B. (2001). Polyunsaturated Fats and Cancer. Second Opinions. http://www.second-opinions.co.uk/fats_and_cancer.html

20 Elwood JM, Jopson J. (1997). Melanoma and sun exposure: an overview of published studies. Int J Cancer. 73(2):198-203.

21 The University of Sydney. (2005). University of Sydney researchers find sunlight may have beneficial effects on cancer. http://www.usyd.edu.au/research/news/2005/feb/02_cancer.shtml

22 Beral, V et al. (1982). Malignant melanoma and exposure to fluorescent lighting at work. Lancet. 2(8293):290-3.

23 White, E, et al. (1994). Case-control study of malignant melanoma in Washington state. Constitutional factors and sun exposure. Am J Epidemiol. 139: 857-868.

24 Elwood, J. (1996). Melanoma and sun exposure. Seminars in Oncology. 23(6): 650-666.

25 Kaskel, P, et al. (2001). Outdoor activities in childhood: a protective factor for cutaneous melanoma? Results of a case-control study in 271 matched pairs. Br J Dermatol. 145(4): 602-9.

26 Danielsson C, et al. (1998). Differential apoptotic response of human mela-noma cells to 1alpha, 25-dihydroxyvitamin D3 and its analogues. *Cell Death Differ.* 5:946.

27 Yudoh K, et al. (1999). 1alpha, 25-dihydroxyvitamin D3 inhibits in vitro in-vasiveness through the extracellular matrix and in vivo pulmonary metastasis of B16 mouse melanoma. *J Lab Clin Med.* 133:120.

28 Black AK, Fincham N, Greaves MW, Hensby CN. Time course changes in levels of arachidonic acid and prostaglandins D2, E2, F2 a in human skin fol-lowing ultraviolet B irradiation. Br J Clin Pharmacol 1980;10:453-7.

29 Harris RB, et al. Fatty acid composition of red blood cell membranes and risk of squamous cell carcinoma of the skin. *Cancer Epidemiol Biomarkers Prev.* 2005 Apr;14(4):906-12.

30 Wilson RB, Hutcheson DP, Wideman L.. Dimethylhydrazine-induced Colon Tumors in Rats Fed Diets Containing Beef Fat or Corn Oil with and without Wheat Bran, Amer J Clin Nutr 30:176, 1977

31 Frei, B. Reactive Oxygen Species and Antioxidant Vitamins. The Linus Pauling Institute.

32 Liu, G. et al. Omega 3 but not omega 6 fatty acids inhibit AP-1 activity and cell transformation in JB6 cells

33 Hipsley, EH. (1974). Malignant melanoma and diet. *Med J Aust.* 1:810.

34 Blot, WJ, et al. Nutrition intervention trials in Linxian, China: supplemen-tation with specific vitamin/mineral combinations, cancer incidence, and disease-specific mortality in the general population. J Natl Cancer Inst. 1993 Sep 15;85(18):1483-92.

35 Lee J, Jiang S, Levine N, Watson RR. Carotenoid supplementation reduces erythema in human skin after simulated solar radiation exposure. Proc Soc Exp Biol Med 2000;223:170-4.

36 Heinrich U, Gartner C, Wiebusch M, et al. Supplementation with b-caro-tene or a similar amount of mixed carotenoids protects humans from UV-induced erythema. J Nutr 2003;133:98-101.

37 Anstey AV. Systemic photoprotection with a-tocopherol (vitamin E) and b-carotene. Clin Exp Dermatol 2002;27:170-6.

38 Stahl W, Sies H. Carotenoids and protection against solar UV radiation. Skin Pharmacol Appl Skin Physiol 2002;15:291-6.

39 Di Mascio et al. 1990, Shimidzu et al. 1996

40 Kurashige et al. 1990

41 http://www.astaxanthin.org/benefits.htm

42 Gradelet, et al., 1998

43 Maduro, R. New scientific evidence continues to demonstrate that the ozone depletion models -and the resulting ban on CFCs- are based on a Big Lie. New Scientific Evidence Proves Ozone Depletion Theory False. http://mitosyfraudes.8k.com/INGLES/Crista.html

44 Scotto Joseph, "Solar Radiation," From the Biostatistics Branch, Division of Cancer Etiology, National Cancer Institute, Bethesda, Maryland

45 Kolata, G. (2005). Melanoma Is Epidemic. Or Is It? Truthout. http://www.truthout.org/issues_05/080905HA.shtml

46 Welch, HG, et al. (2005). Skin biopsy rates and incidence of melanoma: population based ecological study. BMJ. http://bmj.bmjjournals.com/cgi/content/abstract/bmj.38516.649537.E0v1

47 Kolata, Gina. "Melanoma is Epidemic. Or is it?" New York Times. August 9, 2005

48 Berwick M, et al. (2005). Sun exposure and mortality from melanoma. J Natl Cancer Inst. 97(3):195-9.

49 Schroeder, Sarah. "Benchmarks: Background on Skin Cancer," National Cancer Institute. July 1, 2003.

CHAPTER SIX

Sunlight Prevents Seventeen Deadly Cancers

"Ask anyone in America if the sun causes cancer and they will quickly answer yes. Ask them if the sun prevents cancer and they will tell you to see a psychiatrist."

– John Cannell, MD

Y ou've seen that repeated sunburns can contribute to the development the less severe forms of skin cancer, and that regular sensible exposure to sunlight <u>decreases</u> your risk of melanoma. Now we will look at how natural sunlight can <u>save</u> you from many other types of cancer, including breast, prostate and colon cancer.

Staying away from the sun to avoid skin cancer doesn't make sense because it prevents your body from making sufficient vitamin D and raises your

---

The Top 3 Cancers Stopped Cold by Vitamin D

- Breast Cancer
- Colon Cancer
- Ovarian Cancer

---

overall cancer risk. Dr. Edward Giovannucci, a Harvard University professor of medicine and nutrition stated at a lecture to the American Association for Cancer Research that his research suggests adequate vitamin D could prevent up to 30 deaths for every skin cancer death.

"I would challenge anyone to find an area or nutrient or any factor that has such consistent anti-cancer benefits as vitamin D," Giovannucci told the cancer scientists. "The data are really quite remarkable."

More Sunlight Found to Fight Cancer in the Forties

Dr. Frank Apperly discovered that in cities between 10 and 40 degrees latitude there was an 85 percent higher overall cancer death rate than cities farther south. Farther north, in cities between 40 and 50 degrees latitude, there was a 118 percent higher cancer death rate. Going farther north still, in cities between 50 and 60 degrees latitude there was a 150 percent higher death rate from cancer. [1]

Latitude	Overall cancer death rate increase (over farthest southern latitudes)
10 to 40 degrees	85 percent higher
40 to 50 degrees	118 percent higher
50 to 60 degrees	150 percent higher

Dr. Apperly conducted his research in the 1940's. Scientists essentially ignored Dr. Apperly's potentially life saving research until 25 years ago when it was found that rates of breast cancer were twice as high in the Northeast as in the Sun Belt.[2] Only then did researchers begin to understand and acknowledge the connection between sunlight and cancer prevention.

In 1980, Frank and Cedric Garland, epidemiologists and brothers, noticed a similar pattern on maps that showed the geographic incidence of colon cancer. The Garlands and their colleague Edward Gorham were the first to suggest that differing vitamin D levels might account for the variation.

More recently, Dr. William Grant, a former NASA physicist and frequently published vitamin D researcher, focused on the rates of cancer in various parts of the United States in relation to the amount of sunlight the region received. After examining data from 506 regions, he found that cancer mortality increased as levels of exposure to UVB light decreased.

He cited statistics that show as you move farther south in the United States, the death rates for breast, colon, and ovarian cancer significantly decrease. *For example, the breast cancer death rate in the South is approximately half of that in the North and Northeast sections of the country.* Dr. Grant concluded that this is due to the varying levels of vitamin D produced by sunlight. [3]

Sunlight Could Save Thousands – And It's Free!

Sunlight is a powerful healer. Let's put things in perspective:

- Doctors diagnosed 59,600 people with melanoma skin cancer in 2005, according to the American Cancer Society. Melanoma causes the most skin cancer deaths. It accounts for about 7,800 of the total 10,600 skin cancer deaths each year.

- The total number of cancer deaths annually from all kinds of cancer in the U.S. is 570,280.

- *Every year, internal cancers kill 52 times more people than skin cancers!*

- Your risk of dying from melanoma is only a small fraction of your risk from other cancers.

The research shows that simple sun exposure can prevent thousands of these deaths. Now even the mainstream is beginning to listen.

"A balance is required between avoiding an increase in the risk of skin cancer and getting enough ultraviolet radiation exposure to achieve adequate vitamin D levels."

– Australia Cancer Council, "Risks and Benefits of Sun Exposure" March 2005

How Sunlight Dramatically Reduces Cancer Risks

Although researchers have long known that sunlight can prevent cancers, the link between vitamin D and cancer prevention came to light recently. The Journal of *Cancer Research* published a breakthrough study in 1987. Researchers found for the first time ever that vitamin D could stop human cancer cells from growing!

The researchers used vitamin D (specifically calcitriol) to block malignant melanoma tumors from taking hold in human cells. It worked. From their findings, they proposed vitamin D as a potential treatment for melanoma and other cancers. [4] Since then, additional clinical studies have confirmed that vitamin D can in fact inhibit human cancer of the skin, colon, breast, and even blood. [5] [6]

When we examine different groups' risk factors for cancer, we can see that there is a definite connection between conditions that inhibit the body's creation or use of vitamin D and higher cancer rates.

Group	Cancer Risk	Connection to Vitamin D
African Americans	Higher rates of cancer than whites.	More pigment in skin. Need more sunlight to make vitamin D.

Obese	Higher rates of cancer than average	Fat traps vitamin D, causing lower levels circulating in the blood
Diabetics	More prone to cancer	Damaged kidneys have trouble converting vitamin D into a usable form.
Japanese	Overall low cancer rates although their sun exposure is also low	Their diet includes large quantities of fatty fish, rich in vitamin D.

Dr. Gordon Ainsleigh, a sunlight advocate, encourages sunbathing to foster healthy vitamin D levels to fight cancer. In 1992, Ainsleigh reviewed 50 years worth of medical literature on cancer and the sun. He reported in the journal *Preventive Medicine* that widespread regular, moderate sunbathing would lower the incidence of breast and colon cancer death rates by a whopping one-third.[7]

Protect Yourself from 17 Kinds of Cancer

It has been clearly shown that there is an inverse relationship between the incidence of at least 17 different cancers and sun exposure. The more sunlight people get, the lower their risk of developing numerous types of cancer. Breast, colon, and ovarian cancer show the strongest inverse relationship. Sunlight may also reduce the risk of bladder, uterine, pancreatic, esophageal, rectal, and stomach cancers.

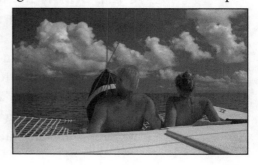

Defeat Breast Cancer with Sunshine

Breast cancer is the most common cancer in women. It claims 370,000 lives worldwide each year. In North America there are 180,000 women diagnosed annually. Like other cancers where sunlight plays a role, the annual death rate for breast cancer varies considerably from region to region.

Breast cancer rates are twice as high in the northeast as they are in the south and southwest. An epidemiological study in 1980 revealed the risk for women who live in areas with less available sunlight is 40 percent higher than for women who live in Hawaii or Florida.[8]

In addition to the geographical distribution data, the clinical data also points to the strong protective role of vitamin D in the incidence of breast cancer. In one study, women in the lowest quartile of serum vitamin D had five times the risk of breast cancer compared with women in the highest quartile.

Clinical studies show the more sunlight you get, the lower your risk of:

- Breast Cancer
- Prostate Cancer
- Colon Cancer
- Ovarian Cancer
- Non-Hodgkin's Lymphoma
- And at least 12 other types of cancer!

Live in a Sunny State and Lower Your Breast Cancer Risk

If you call a sunny state home, you cut your risk for breast cancer by more than half. According to research at the Northern California Cancer Center there's a… "25 percent to 65 percent reduction in breast cancer risk among women whose longest residence was in a state with high solar radiation."[9] We know conclusively from clinical studies like these that breast cancer is lower in areas with more UVB radiation and *higher* in areas with less sunlight.

Women who work outside have a far lower rate of breast cancer. A recent study by the National Cancer Institute reveals women whose jobs

require consistent sun exposure are less likely to die of breast cancer.[10] If you look at the research, some 45,000 to 117,000 US women could potentially avoid breast cancer just by getting a moderate dose of daily sunlight!

Vitamin D: Your Natural Breast Cancer Protection

Clinical studies at St. George's Hospital in London tell us a lot. Doctors there have found that breast tissue produces its own activated vitamin D (calcitriol). They hypothesize that this is for disease protection. There's a catch, though: the pre-hormone vitamin D must be circulating in the blood or breast tissue to create activated vitamin D. The same researchers also found that women with the lowest vitamin D levels have five times the risk of developing breast cancer.[11]

Reduce Your Prostate Cancer Risk with More Time in the Sun

Doctors diagnose approximately 185,000 men with prostate cancer every year in the United States. More than 30,000 of them die from the disease. Rates continue to rise. Doctors estimate that one in six men will be diagnosed with prostate cancer during their lifetime.

For years, doctors never made the connection between sunlight and prostate cancer. Then Professor Gary Schwartz, Ph.D., of Wake Forest University's School of Medicine made a connection.

In 1990, he noticed that the populations who get too little vitamin D are the same populations who get the most prostate cancer. He found that there was a strong north-south trend in the disease, just like in rickets. Schwartz concluded that men living in sun-drenched southern climates were 20-40 percent less likely to get prostate cancer than their northern counterparts.[12]

Ongoing research backs him up:

1. Many scientists are beginning to believe that *vitamin D deficiency is the number one cause of prostate cancer!* Prostate cancer patients regularly exhibit a vitamin D deficiency.[13]

2. A recent study by the National Cancer Institute confirms that people in the sunniest places get less prostate cancer. Men with the highest sun exposure have up to 50 percent less risk than those with the lowest sun exposure.[14]

3. Vitamin D inhibits the growth of prostate cancer cells and triggers their death. With sufficient vitamin D from cod liver oil or sunlight, fewer men would experience prostate cancer.

Many doctors believe that African-American men are predisposed to prostate cancer. And considering that they are 65 percent more likely to be diagnosed and have twice the risk of dying from it than white males, this seems to make sense. But the truth is that their risk has nothing to do with a genetic predisposition.

The increased risk of prostate cancer in black men is strongly related to their vitamin D status. This is evidenced by the fact that black men in the northern U.S., Canada and the UK are experiencing rapidly rising rates of prostate cancer. While on the other hand, black men in the Caribbean and Africa in particular, have much lower rates of the disease.

Prostate cancer effects almost 200,000 men each year in the U.S. alone. But research shows that with adequate vitamin D 37,000 to 74,000 men in the US alone would not have to endure this disease.

Save Yourself from the Second Deadliest Cancer in the U.S.

Colon cancer is the second leading cause of cancer death in the United States following lung cancer. An estimated 145,290 new cases of colon cancer were diagnosed in the United States in 2005. Sadly, doctors estimate that 56,295 of those will die from the disease.

Research on vitamin D and sunlight gives us promising new information that can help us turn the tide on this disease. Like breast and prostate cancer, colon cancer is more common at higher latitudes where there is less sunlight. Scientists now believe vitamin D levels are the reason.

In a study published in the *Lancet* in 1989, researchers at the University of California School of Medicine took blood samples from 25,000 volunteers over an eight-year period. The group with the highest circulating vitamin D levels showed an 80-percent reduction in their risk of colon cancer.[15] The researchers concluded that vitamin D could in fact protect against colon cancer.

Another study by Dr. Edward Gorham at the Naval Health Research Center in San Diego showed that people who have good vitamin D levels have lower risks for colon cancer. Dr. Gorham reviewed evidence collected from 1,400 individuals through five different studies and concluded that people who got the equivalent of 1,000 to 2,000 IU of vitamin D daily were 50% less like get colon cancer.

Sunlight... A Cancer-Fighting Miracle

Lung Cancer

Tests show that UV radiation helps prevent the leading cause of cancer death in the United States – lung cancer. Scientists bred mice specifically to develop lung cancer. They then exposed some of these mice to UV radiation. Others not receiving UV exposure acted as the control group. The mice exposed to UV radiation developed less lung cancer than those who didn't get the UV light exposure.[16]

Non-Hodgkin's Lymphoma (NHL)

For some time, researchers believed that sun exposure was behind the rising rates non-Hodgkin's lymphoma, a deadly cancer of the blood. Yet a study that was designed to confirm sunlight as a risk factor for NHL found just the opposite to be true.

The researchers analyzed the personal histories of 704 NHL patients and compared them to the personal histories of a control group. They found that greater cumulative sun exposure reduced relative risk for the disease by up to 35%.[17]

An additional study helps confirm these findings. In this case-controlled study, researchers found that sunbathing reduced NHL risk.[18] Researchers suggest that vitamin D is the likely reason for these findings. In addition to its affects on other cancer cells, vitamin D supports the immune system, from which NHL cancers arise.

Vitamin D's 7 Keys to Cancer Prevention

1. Converts tumor cells into normal cells
2. Prevents cancer cells from multiplying and tells them when to die
3. Keeps cancer from spreading
4. Suppresses genes responsible for cell proliferation
5. Inhibits formation of new blood vessels
6. Moderates immune responsiveness
7. Increases the oxygen-carrying capacity of the blood

Spark Your Own Vitamin D Production to Trigger Multiple Cancer-Fighting Actions

Now that it's been shown *that* sunlight prevents cancer, let's examine *how* this happens. Sunlight sparks your body's ability to make vitamin D. This vitamin, or hormone, has seven essential actions in your body that are key to reducing your risk of many different types of cancer.

Healthy cells exist in a balance between new cell creation and cell death. When a cell is out of balance it loses control of these natural processes. A cancerous tumor starts when a cell with damaged DNA replicates instead of self-destructing. Vitamin D helps to regulate this process, keeping cells in their proper balance.

1. **Vitamin D converts tumor cells into normal cells** – The cells in your body go through an organized process to duplicate themselves. This constant state of renewal is how your body remains healthy and strong. Each cell is duplicated or "differentiated" for a unique purpose. Some become lung cells, others skin cells, some liver cells, and so on.

Why is this important? Because cancer cells start out the same way. They divide rapidly but don't differentiate themselves into specific cells. Vitamin D helps with cell differentiation. By helping cancers replicate into specific cells, vitamin D can help restore these cells to productivity and inhibit cancer growth.

2. **Vitamin D prevents cancer cells from multiplying and tells them when to die** – Laboratory and animal studies show that vitamin D prevents cancer cells from multiplying and also tells them when to die. This is called "apoptosis," or programmed cell death. Two colleagues at Roswell Park Cancer Institute in New York showed that cancer cells can't reproduce and spread to new tissue when introduced to vitamin D.[19]

3. **Vitamin D keeps cancer from spreading** – Since vitamin D promotes normal cell growth, it helps to prevent cancerous cells from spreading. Drug companies are attempting to create synthetic forms of vitamin D for anti-cancer therapy.[20]

4. **Vitamin D suppresses genes responsible for cell proliferation** – Laboratory research shows that vitamin D can suppress genes prone to mutation. In one study, vitamin D receptor genes bound p53 genes, which are likely to mutate and form cancerous growths.[21]

5. **Vitamin D inhibits formation of new blood vessels that feed tumors** – The creation of new blood vessels in your body is called angiogenesis. During this process, blood vessels begin to sprout off of existing vessels. This is fine unless you're talking about cancer. For a tumor to have any chance of growing, there must be formation of new blood vessels to feed its high metabolism.

Sunlight Prevents Seventeen Deadly Cancers

This is why pharmaceutical companies have made much ado about drugs that can inhibit angiogenesis to cancerous tumors. Vitamin D does this naturally. Studies at Harvard Medical School show that vitamin D is a potent inhibitor of the creation of undesirable new blood vessels that supply tumors with nutrients.[22]

6. **Vitamin D moderates immune responsiveness** – Vitamin D works with the immune system to keep it functioning smoothly. In the face of a cancerous tumor, vitamin D can help to step up immune response and break the body's tolerance of a tumor. In other words, it signals the body to attack the tumor.[23]

7. **Vitamin D increases the oxygen-carrying capacity of the blood** – Vitamin D increases the oxygen content of your blood as well as the capacity of blood to deliver oxygen to the tissues.[24] [25] This is important for a healthy body in many ways, but when it comes to avoiding cancer, it's essential. A high oxygen environment kills cancer and a low oxygen environment breeds cancer.

Designing Cancer-Killers

Have you heard of what could be one of the biggest breakthroughs in cancer treatment? Researchers from the National Cancer Institute have been able to genetically change a patient's cells to battle cancer cells.

Researchers have been working on this one for years. In a study published in the journal Science, researchers have documented that their genetically-engineered cells have cured two patients of a deadly form of skin cancer, melanoma, which had spread throughout their bodies. Even though researchers caution that the long-term success of this treatment is yet unknown, they remain cautiously optimistic that this can applied to various cancers.

Dr. Otto Warburg discovered this in 1931 and won his first Nobel Prize for his study called, *Prime Cause and Prevention of Cancer.* Dr. Warburg proved that cancer is caused by a lack of oxygen respiration in cells. Normal cells meet their energy needs by using oxygen. Cancer cells meet their energy needs, at least in part, by the fermentation of sugar instead.

Oxygen: Lethal to Cancer

High oxygen levels are extremely lethal to cancer tissue, but don't harm normal cells. Cancer simply cannot handle a high oxygen environment.

Lack of exercise, the foods you eat, toxins in the body, or reduced circulation can all result in a low oxygen environment.

A word for the wise – If you want to prevent cancer, get as much oxygen in your body as you can – exercise, detoxify your body and get outdoors – for both the fresh air and to enjoy the sunlight.

Surprising Success of Sunlight in Surviving Cancer

If vitamin D created by sunlight prevents cancer, could it help patients who already have cancer? Despite the logic to this hypothesis to date there are few studies on the treatment of cancer with vitamin D.

There is much anecdotal evidence though. Like Dr. Zane Kime's case involving one of his patients with breast cancer whom he encouraged to sunbathe and to eat a whole food diet with no refined vegetable oils. Within months, the patient recovered and experienced no remission in the following years.[26]

Sunlight Prevents Seventeen Deadly Cancers

Reinhold Vieth, a vitamin D expert at the University of Toronto, gave 2,000 units of vitamin D to men with advanced prostate cancer. The treatment resulted in a measurable improvement in the PSA scores for a majority of the men. PSA is a marker used to evaluate the spread of prostate cancer.[27]

There are currently a number of researchers, including Dr. Johan Moan, Ph.D., who are doing cutting edge work on the study of cancer survival as related to vitamin D status.

One study, from the Harvard School of Public Health, found that lung cancer patients, who underwent surgery in the summer and had the highest blood levels of vitamin D, had a 72 percent chance of surviving the next five years, while those that had their operations in the winter and had the lowest vitamin D levels only had a 30 percent five-year survival.

A few in modern medicine are using UV light to treat some forms of cancer. Dr. Andrew Weil writes that:

> *"Ultraviolet blood irradiation is used in both conventional and alternative medicine for different reasons. In conventional medicine, UV blood irradiation... is an FDA-approved treatment for cutaneous T-cell lymphoma (a type of cancer affecting the skin) as well as for psoriasis..."* [28]

In *Light: Medicine of the Future*, Dr. Jacob Liberman describes photodynamic therapy where cancerous cells are targeted with red laser light as "precise like a laser." Unlike imprecise chemotherapy and surgery, this readily available therapy is simple, painless, and has a higher degree of success treating local cancers than conventional treatments.[29]

Tips to Enjoying the Cancer Fighting Benefits of Sunshine

Sunlight is life saving, and it does far more to prevent cancer than cause it. Here are five steps to get sun safely, improve your health and reduce your risk of deadly cancers:

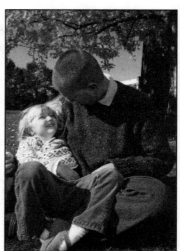

1. **A little sun goes a long way** – At the right time of day and year, it takes very little time in the sun to maximize the benefits to your health. At high noon on a summer's day, you can get a full daily dose of vitamin D in as little as ten minutes depending on your coloring.

2. **Obey the laws of good nutrition** – Watch your diet and eat whole foods, not refined ones. Get plenty of high quality lean protein from sources like grass-fed beef, wild Alaskan salmon, sardines, eggs, and chicken. Also eat plenty of fruit and vegetables. These foods not only boost your body's natural defenses against cancer, they also help repair any minor sun damage that your skin may experience. You'll see more specific foods to eat later in this chapter.

3. **Don't ever let your skin burn** – You should get sun gradually and consistently over a long period of time. If you are sensitive to sun, you may start out by only exposing small parts of your body, and building up to more exposure. Never allow your skin to burn.

   Most people get sunburned because they are so eager for a tan they overdo it. Don't ever bake in the heat, and never spend too long in the sun at one time. Frequent short exposures produce much better results for your health than prolonged exposure. If practical, you should spend a few minutes in the sun each day, several times a day.

4. **Know your skin type** – If you have very fair skin and burn easily, you have a higher risk of skin cancer. Even so, it is safe to be in the sun, as long as you don't overdo it. If you have darker skin, you'll need to increase the duration of your exposure to get the full benefits of vitamin D production – see the following chart for different skin types. Gauge your sun exposure accordingly.

Skin Type	Sun History	Example
I	Always burns easily, never tans, extremely sun sensitive skin	Red-headed, freckles, Irish/Scots/Welsh
II	Always burns easily, tans minimally, very sun sensitive skin	Fair-skinned, fair-haired, blue-eyed Caucasians
III	Sometimes burns, tans gradually to light brown, sun sensitive skin	Average skin

IV	Burns minimally, always tans to moderate brown, minimally sun sensitive	Mediterranean-type Caucasians
V	Rarely burns, tans well, sun insensitive skin	Middle Eastern, some Hispanics, some African-Americans
VI	Never burns, deeply pigmented, sun insensitive skin	African-American

5. **Skip the chemical sunscreens** – Sunscreen prevents the formation of vitamin D. It also uses chemicals that may not be good for you. We'll look at alternatives in chapter 15.

By using your common sense, you can take full advantage of the healthful benefits of sunlight without damaging your skin or increasing your risks of superficial skin cancers.

Beat Cancer with Nutrition

You can boost the effectiveness of vitamin D and go further toward preventing cancer by giving your body a nutritional cancer-fighting boost. Remember, vitamin D fights cancer in seven ways. Two of those ways – increased immune responsiveness and programmed cell death – are very dependent on certain nutrients in your diet.

Enhance your immune system
A strong immune system is your best defense against cancer. Add these immune-enhancing foods, herbs and supplements to your diet to keep cancers from developing in your body or on your skin.

- **Whey Isolate** – As an addition to smoothies or simply by consuming with water, this milk isolate is well known for its immune boosting properties – especially when it comes to fighting cancer. The essential amino acids and proteins found within whey isolate exert an inhibitory effect on the development of several types of cancers.

- **Selenium** – Studies show that people who are deficient in selenium are more susceptible to viruses and many types of cancer. (Viruses also readily mutate in selenium-deficient individuals.) This mineral is scarce in the food supply. Brazil nuts are the richest natural source.

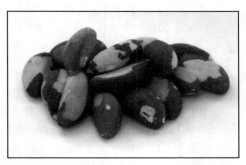

- **Astragalus** – The best-known immune-boosting herb in Chinese medicine, research now shows that astragalus increases the production of Natural Killer cells and lymphocytes.

- **Reishi mushrooms** – The Chinese refer to these as "the mushrooms of immortality." They are widely recognized for their immune boosting and anti-cancer properties.

- **Beta glucan** – Hundreds of studies have shown that this substance, derived from yeast and mushrooms, stimulates the production and activity of immune cells.

Kill Cancerous Cells Naturally
When a cell becomes cancerous, it is supposed to self-destruct. Unfortunately, sometimes something goes awry with the process and cancer cells proliferate. Taking a daily dose of vitamin C and

eating berries regularly can help your body keep its natural pro-grammed cell death process working properly.

- **Vitamin C** – This antioxidant vitamin is wildly successful at helping healthy cells survive while initiating suicide among cancerous ones. Cancer cells need iron to survive and vitamin C helps to prevent the uptake of iron.[30] Iron greedy cancer cells commit suicide during the iron deficiency while healthy, not-so-demanding cells survive.

- **Ellagic Acid** - Bring on the berries! Ellagic acid is found primarily in fruits and nuts, like grapes, pomegranate, red raspberry, strawberry, blueberry, pecans and walnuts. Ellagic acid causes apoptosis in cancer cells in the laboratory. In addition to inducing apoptosis among cancer cells it also surrounds cellular DNA to serve as a shield. Amazingly, ellagic acid protects the genetic blue print of a cell by shielding it from damaging free radicals! It is a proven anti-carcinogen, anti-mutagen, and anticancer initiator. Because ellagic acid is concentrated in the seeds, you should chew berry until you feel the crunch, or use a juicer. Black and red raspberries, blackberries, marionberries, loganberries, and strawberries are especially good sources ellagic acid. Pomegranate extracts are widely available as nutritional supplements with high ellagic acid content. Topical ellagic acid is especially promising for skin cancer treatment and prevention. If you want to try this use pomegranate extract in capsules, open the capsules and mix with aloe vera gel.

Finally, you can help your body keep cancers from getting a foothold by eating more antioxidant rich foods. Antioxidants help the body clean up free radicals that can damage a cell's DNA giving cancer a start. Use this table, "The Top Ten Antioxidant Rich Foods" to choose foods that give your body a diverse number of powerful antioxidants.

The Top Ten Antioxidant Rich Foods

Food	Antioxidant Punch
Berries – Blueberries, Strawberries, Blackberries, etc.	Proanthocyandins and ellagic acid fight cancer, heart disease, and cognitive decline.
Cruciferous Vegetables – Broccoli, Cauliflower, Asparagus, etc.	Indole-3-Carbinol and beta carotene help balance hormones and fight cancer.
Tomatoes	Lycopene and glutathione fight cancer and boost the immune system. The skin uses lycopene to make repairs to UV damaged skin.
Red Grapes	Resveratrol scavenges free radicals and reduces systemic inflammation.
Garlic	A broad range of antioxidants that reduce inflammation, fight aging, and prevent heart disease and cancer.
Dark Leafy Greens – Spinach, Kale, Swiss Chard, etc.	Lutien, vitamin C, and beta carotene all fight free radicals and help protect delicate tissues from cell damage.
Oranges	Vitamin C helps build healthy collagen.
Green Tea	Catechins fight cancer and reduce inflammation.
Olive oil	A broad range of antioxidants plus monounsaturated fats which help to fight inflammation and cellular damage.
Cocoa	Flavanols in high quality cocoas protect the skin and improve its appearance.

Remember, fear of skin cancer isn't a good reason to shut out the sun. Sunshine helps prevent the most deadly type of skin cancer (melanoma) and many other kinds of cancer. And, other types of cancers kill 52 times more people than skin cancer.

In the next chapter, we'll look at the connection between sunshine and the youthful, radiant and healthy appearance of your skin including the recent concern over "photoaging".

(Endnotes)

1 Hobday, R. (1999). *The Healing Sun: Sunlight and Health in the 21st Century.* Scotland: Findhorn Press. p. 67.

2 John EM, Schwartz GG, et al. "Vitamin D and Breast Cancer Risk: The NHANES I Epidemiologic Follow-up Study, 1971–1975 to 1992," *Cancer Epidem Bio & Prev* 1999; 8: 399-406

3 Grant, W. (2002). *Cancer.* 94:1867-75.

4 Eisman JA, et al. (1987). Suppression of in vivo growth of human cancer solid tumor xenografts by 1,25-dihydroxyvitamin D3. *Cancer Res.* 47:21.

5 Manolagas, SC. (1987). Vitamin D and its relevance to cancer. *Anticancer Res.* 7:625.

6 DeLuca HF, Ostrem V. (1986). The Relationship between the Vitamin D System and Cancer. *Adv Exp Med Biol.* 206:413.

7 Hobday, R. (1999). *The Healing Sun: Sunlight and Health in the 21st Century.* Scotland: Findhorn Press. p. 67.

8 Hobday, R. (1999). *The Healing Sun: Sunlight and Health in the 21st Century.* Scotland: Findhorn Press. p. 70.

9 John, EM, et al. (1999). Vitamin D and breast cancer risk: the NHANES I Epidemiologic follow-up study, 1971-1975 to 1992. National Health and Nutrition Examination Survey. *Cancer Epidemiol Biomarkers Prev.* 8(5):399-406.

10 Freedman MD, et al. "Sunlight and mortality from breast, ovarian, colon, prostate, and non-melanoma skin cancer: a composite death certificate based case-control study," *Occup and Environ Med* 2002; 59: 257-62

11 Lowe LC, et al. (2005). Plasma 25-hydroxy vitamin D concentrations, vitamin D receptor genotype and breast cancer risk in a UK Caucasian population. *Eur J Cancer.* 41(8):1164-9. Epub 2005 Apr 14.

12 Hanchette, CL, Schwartz GG. (1992). Geographic patterns of prostate cancer mortality. Evidence for a protective effect of ultraviolet radiation. *Cancer.* 70(12):2861-9.

13 Luscombe, CJ, et al. (2001). Exposure to ultra-violet radiation: association with susceptibility and age at presentation with prostate cancer. *Lancet.* 358: 641-2.

14 Luscombe, CJ, et al. (2001). Exposure to ultra-violet radiation: association with susceptibility and age at presentation with prostate cancer. *Lancet.* 358: 641-2.

15 Garland, CF, et al. (1989). Serum 25-hydroxyvitamin D and colon cancer: eight-year prospective study. *Lancet.* 2(8673):1176-8.

16 Kime, ZR. (1980). *Sunlight.* Penryn, CA: World Health Publications. p. 111

17 Hughes AM, et al. "Sun exposure may protect against non-Hodgkin lymphoma: a case-control study," *Int J Cancer* 2004; 112(5): 865-71

18 The University of Sydney. (2005). Researchers find sunlight may have beneficial effects on cancer.
http://www.usyd.edu.au/research/news/2005/feb/02_cancer.shtml

19 http://www.spiritualityhealth.com/newsh/items/article/item_6501.html

20 Studzinski GP, Moore DC. (1996). Vitamin D and the retardation of tumor progression. In Watson RR, Mufti SI, editors, Nutrition and cancer. Boca Raton: CRC Press. p. 257-82.

21 Maruyama R, et al. "Comparative genome analysis identifies the vitamin D receptor gene as a direct target of p53-mediated transcriptional activation." *Cancer Res* 2006; 66(9): 4574-83

22 Shokravi MT, et al. (1995). Vitamin D inhibits angiogenesis in transgenic murine retinoblastoma. *Inv Oph*. 36:83.

23 Adorini L, et al. "Vitamin d receptor agonists, cancer and the immune system: an intricate relationship." *Curr Top Med Chem* 2006; 6(12): 1297-1301

24 Miley, G. (1944). The Present Status of Ultraviolet Blood Irradiation. *Arch Phys Ther*. 25:357.

25 Wiesner, S. (1973). The Influence of Ultraviolet Light on the Oxygen Uptake of the Tissues in Arterial Occlussive Diseases, Radiobiol Radiothere Vol. 14.

26 Hobday, R. (1999). *The Healing Sun: Sunlight and Health in the 21st Century.* Scotland: Findhorn Press. p. 75.

27 Vieth R, Woo TC, et al. "Pilot study: potential role of vitamin D (Cholecalciferol) in patients with PSA relapse after definitive therapy," *Nutr Cancer* 2005; 51(1): 32-36

28 Weil, A. (2002). Can Light Cure Disease? Does the alternative medicine treatment called ultraviolet blood irradiation have any validity whatsoever? Weil. http://www.drweil.com/app/cda/drw_cda.html-command=TodayQA-questionId=98869

29 Dougherty, TJ. (1989). Photoradiation Therapy – New Approaches. *Seminars in Surgical Oncology*. 5:6-16.

30 Kang, JS et al. (2005) Sodium ascorbate (vitamin C) induces apoptosis in melanoma cells via the down-regulation of transferrin receptor dependent iron uptake. *J Cell Physiol*. 204(1):192-7.

CHAPTER SEVEN

Keeping Your Skin Youthful

"Only in the last few decades, has the accelerated aging of the skin become so noticeable, especially since Americans have increased their intake of polyunsaturated fat. This increase of polyunsaturated fat has been in the form of refined oils and not in the natural food products that contain polyunsaturated fats."

– Zane Kime, Sunlight

You have seen that the sun does not cause, and actually protects you from, lethal cancers. But the appearance of your skin is a common concern with sun exposure. What about aging of your skin? Skin exposed to UV light regularly for longer periods may develop increased freckles and wrinkles and succumb to changes recently termed "photoaging".

You may be surprised to know that **research does link moderate sun exposure to premature skin aging.**

Like skin cancer, managing skin aging is much more complex that avoiding our native sun. The sun is

What is Photoaging?

We use the term photoaging to describe damage done to the skin from over exposure to ultraviolet radiation. The signs are wrinkles, increased freckling, irregular brown spots, surface roughness and pigmentation changes that are not part of the normal aging process. Research links both inflammation and a breakdown of connective tissue and collagen in the skin to photoaging.

merely one of many contributing co-factors in photoaging – and there is more to skin aging and appearance than just photoaging.

In fact, smart exposure to the sun, with a few caveats, can actually help keep your skin looking healthier and younger – and, you'll reap the many natural health benefits.

The Causes of Old-Looking Skin

It is worth knowing the factors that can damage your skin causing it to lose its tone and wrinkle earlier than you'd like. Then, you'll know action you can take to keep your skin taut and healthy while still taking advantage of the benefits of sunlight.

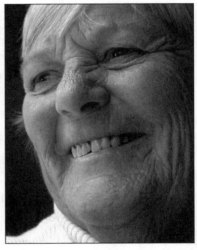

Some of the big contributors to damaged skin include overexposure to sunlight, nutritional deficiencies, over consumption of artificial polyunsaturated fats, inadequate consumption of omega-3 fats, exposure to toxins and allergens in our food and drink, air pollution, chemical lotions and creams, and smoking. Let's take a closer look at each of these factors.

Does Sunlight Damage
Your Skin's Appearance?

People slather up with sunscreen and head into intense sun for hours thinking they're safe from overexposure to the sun. You've already seen why that idea is false when it comes to skin cancer. The practice is equally ineffective when it comes to skin aging.

Most sunscreens block UV-B light, the light that causes sunburn. But most do not block UV-A light, and it is overexposure to UV-A light which accelerates photoaging of your skin. When you spend a long time in the sun, unprotected from UV-A, this type of radiation can chemically transform and excite certain acids in your skin that then contribute to photoaging pigmentation changes and wrinkles.[1]

Even worse, many sunscreens still use a compound called PABA. This chemical actually increases photoaging because it inhibits your skin's ability to repair cellular damage. And there is another reason you should avoid PABA: Many people are allergic and get a rash which looks like a sunburn and further inflames and damages skin.

Overexposure to sunlight can also generate free radicals that can damage skin cells and reduce the amount of antioxidants present in your skin, specifically vitamin C, vitamin E, and CoQ10.[2]

Reverse the Effects of aging with three powerful nutrients:

- Vitamin C – 1000 mg
- CoQ10 – 100 mg
- Vitamin E – 400 I.U.
- Mixed Tocopherols

The effect of sunlight on the antioxidants present in the skin is important. While moderate sun exposure actually helps to increase antioxidants present in the skin, inappropriate ratios of UV-A radiation or overexposure consumes and lowers antioxidant levels in your skin. This tells us in part how sunlight can damage your skin… and it helps us find ways to counteract the process.

Your body uses vitamin C to make collagen. Collagen forms a

kind of latticework or scaffolding as the basis of your skin's structure. When you have healthy collagen, you have taunt, smooth and toned skin. When any factor damages your skin's collagen, your skin loses its scaffolding, sags and begins to wrinkle. With a deficiency of vitamin C, this process goes on unchecked without repair.

Additionally, vitamin C is critical to many of your skin's other maintenance and repair processes. When your skin lacks adequate vitamin C, these processes are retarded, slowing repair and contributing to aging of your skin. Later in this chapter, you'll find out how to restore vitamin C in the skin and reverse this feature of aging to help your skin stay healthier and more youthful looking.

The Foods You Eat Affect Your Skin… for Better or Worse

While photoaging can play a part in the appearance of your skin, it is complicated by a number of factors. If you take good care of your skin, you are less likely to experience sun-related damage. And by giving your skin the nutrients it needs to make immediate repairs against sun damage, you'll be able to spend adequate time in the sun and have the capacity to replenish antioxidants and make the repairs needed for a more youthful, fresher and more radiant look to your skin.

Research reported in the *American Journal of Clinical Nutrition* found that people with lower micronutrient and fatty acid levels experience skin aging at a faster rate than those with higher levels of these nutrients.[3] Many other studies have confirmed that nutrition plays a strong role in both skin aging and increased formation of wrinkles.[4] This only makes sense but has been completely neglected in the modern approach to skin care.

To maintain good tone and texture and keep up your skin's defenses against damage and aging; you must give your skin the right nutrients it needs to make repairs.

A diet rich in a variety of colorful fruits and vegetables is a great first step toward keeping your skin healthy. This is because colorful fruits and vegetables are rich in a variety of antioxidants that help prevent free radicals from damaging your collagen.

Another factor in skin aging is inflammation. Low levels of inflammation either from topical irritants that your skin encounters or from the foods you eat can create a spiral of damage in the skin. An initial small level of inflammation can trigger more inflammation and can eventually disrupt your body's ability to organize collagen into the proper supportive structure for the skin.[5] The result is thinning, sagging skin and wrinkles.

Dietary omega-6 fatty acids from vegetable oils are particularly apt to cause inflammation that will lead to wrinkles when you consume them in excess.

Epidemiological studies of humans on the molecular level show that we need as much omega-3 as omega-6 fatty acids or about a one-to-one ratio. Yet the average American consumes about 16 times more omega-6 fatty acids than omega-3 fatty acids. This imbalance leads inflammation throughout your body.[6]

Processed foods, vegetable oils and grain-fed red meats are the main source of omega-6s in your diet.

At the end of this chapter, you'll find more information on the foods you should eat to boost your levels of wrinkle-fighting antioxidants and lower your body's levels of inflammation.

How You Can Fight Environmental Skin Damage

Common air pollutants also cause problems for your skin. This is partly because of the ability of air pollutants to reduce the amount of vitamin E, a powerful oil-soluble antioxidant, in your skin.[7]

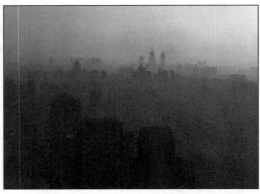

You can counteract the affects of pollution to some degree by keeping your skin clean. Each day you should wash your face both in the morning and in the evening. Choose a gentle, hypo-allergenic cleanser and use it everyday. Everyone's skin is different, so it may take some trial and error to find a cleanser that works well with your skin, but it is worth the effort.

Another form of air pollution that is most damaging to your skin is cigarette smoke. Pollutants in cigarette smoke literally attack your skin. They cause irritation, inflammation, small blood vessel damage, reduced blood flow and repair, stymie normal skin maintenance, lower nutrient levels, cause increased free radical damage, and interfere with normal pigmentation resulting in wrinkled, aged, discoloring and diseased skin.[8] Skin in this weakened and diseased state then becomes "a sitting duck" for any other stressor including even normal sun exposure.

If you live in the city, if you are a smoker, or live with a smoker, your skin is under daily attack. Aside from cleaning it each day, you should take particular care to provide it with extra doses of the nutrients it needs to protect and repair itself. See the section at the

Keeping Your Skin Youthful

end of this chapter for more about foods, supplements, and lotions that can help, protect, soothe, and heal your skin.

Use Good Health to Protect Your Skin and Give it Youthful Glow

Slathering on sunscreen from morning to night will not really protect your skin and it can't give it a healthy appearance. Your body comes equipped with its own skin maintenance and repair systems. One of the best things you can do for youthful, healthy appearing skin is to improve your general health and vigor. Common sense health improving strategies can go a long way to protect your skin from all the factors of aging.

- **Exercise** – Living an active lifestyle gives you overall health benefits, but maybe you didn't realize it benefits the health of your skin, too. By exercising every day, you keep your blood pumping, which brings oxygen to your skin and helps your skin remove toxins that can cause damage if left to accumulate. Regular exercise also helps your body to make collagen, which supports the skin and prevents wrinkles.

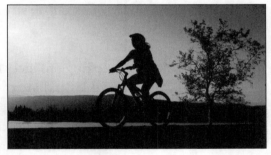

  Chose a variety of exercise for your daily life including: walking, stretching, strength training, and heart-pumping challenges to your aerobic capacity to give your skin the most benefit.

- **Reduce Stress** – Stress contributes to a variety of ailments by reducing your immunity. When you experience stress – especially long term stress – your body reacts by producing the hormones cortisol and adrenaline. Think back to a stressful event in your youth… you may have had an accompanying acne breakout. That's because stress hormones shut down repair and maintenance, letting bacteria and toxins accumulate taking their toll on your skin.

By managing stress and anxiety, you may also benefit your skin. Try breathing deeply when you are faced with a stressful situation. Take time out to pamper yourself – a nice luxurious bath (add a little vitamin E oil for added skin benefit!) or a massage are nice things to do for yourself and your skin. If you're dealing with ongoing stress, join a yoga class – it may help you deal with stress more positively.

Meditation is also good for dealing with stress and may even reduce your body's production of free radicals, which would reduce the amount of oxidative stress your body – and skin – has to deal with.[9]

- **Quit Smoking** – Smoking produces free radicals that accelerate how fast you get wrinkles and increases your risk of melanoma and non-melanoma skin cancers. It also increases the toxins your skin is exposed to, can cause skin discoloration, and increases the overall levels of inflammation in your body. But it doesn't stop there. Smoking causes poor wound healing and an increased risk of scarring, hair loss, psoriasis, and lesions.

If you're a smoker the first step you can take to improve the look and health of your skin is to stop smoking. It's a difficult thing to do, so don't be afraid to seek help. It's one of the best decisions you'll ever make.

- **Drink Lots of Water** – Water is a natural moisturizer, hydrating your skin from the inside out. It's a good idea to test your water for contaminants, and if appropriate, to use a filter.

- **Control Your Exposure** – You need the effects of the sun. But you don't have to overexpose your face. Because we have all started wearing clothing over most of our bodies most of the time, our face, neck and hands get an overexposure relative to the rest of our skin.

  If you are worried about the sun aging your face, then wear a hat. Enjoy 10 or 15 minutes of direct sun exposure because it's good for your eyes, skin, and health, but then cover up the sensitive and overexposed areas. That's all it takes to safely enjoy the sun without using chemical sunscreens.

Four Important Ways to Protect and Nourish Your Skin

Lifestyle changes will go a long way to keep your skin young looking and healthy, but the most important thing you can do for your skin is to nourish it inside and out.

You nourish your skin from the inside by picking foods that are rich in antioxidants that your skin needs to renew itself and repair damage. You nourish your skin from the outside with topical moisturizers that keep it soft and hydrated and that also supply it with nutrients it needs.

The best foods for your skin:

By eating the right kinds of foods, you take care of your skin from the inside out. You should give your skin the tools it needs to constantly renew itself, keeping its toned, youthful look.

Get Your Vitamins Naturally From the Foods You Eat	
Food	**Vitamin Levels**
Citrus Fruit – oranges, grapefruit, tangerines, etc.	Up to 70 mg/serving of vitamin C – builds collagen, reduces inflammation, protects cells.
Cantaloupe	29 mg/serving of vitamin C
Guava	165 mg/serving of vitamin C
Kiwifruit	162 mg/serving of vitamin C
Eggs	140 micrograms (mcg)/serving of vitamin A – powerful antioxidant that helps maintain healthy cells.
Plain Yogurt	35 mcg/serving of vitamin A
Chicken Liver	11,000 mcg/serving of vitamin A
Almonds	11 IU/serving of vitamin E – beneficial to skin health, prevents skin cell damage
Peanut Butter	6 IU/serving of vitamin E
Cooked Spinach	2.5 IU/serving of vitamin E
Beef	3.4 mg/serving of Coenzyme Q10 – an important antioxidant and a building block of the body's tissues.
Sardines	7.3 mg/serving of CoQ10

You need to eat foods rich in the antioxidant vitamins E, C, and A.[10] But don't stop there. Antioxidants are more complicated than you may realize. Aside from these major antioxidants, fruits and vegetables are rich in flavonoids and phytonutrients that also play an antioxidant role. To get the most benefit eat a wide variety of colorful fresh fruits and vegetables and other anti-oxidant rich foods.

For example, in one study, researchers examined the affect of cocoa on skin health after sun exposure. Women consumed cocoa powder rich in flavanols (the cocoa was mixed with water) every day. After 12 weeks, the researchers exposed selected areas of skin to UV rays. Compared with a control group, the women experienced 25% less skin damage. More blood also flowed to the skin tissues boosting skin density and hydration, too.[11]

Use the chart "The Top Ten Antioxidant Rich Foods" found in the previous chapter to help you choose foods that will boost your antioxidants levels.

Take care to reduce the processed foods in your diet. These foods are high in inflammatory vegetable oils that will damage your skin. Most processed foods are also void of nutrients, so you do your skin a double disservice when you eat them.

All foods have either a positive or negative inflammatory affect on your body. You can help improve the quality and health of your skin by choosing more foods that have an anti-inflammatory affect and using inflammatory foods sparingly. In general refined and processed foods trigger an inflammatory reaction while whole, fresh foods or foods rich in omega-3 fatty acids of monounsaturated fats are anti-inflammatory.

In her book, *The Inflammation Free Diet Plan*, Monica Reinagel gives foods an inflammation rating. If they are neutral, they get a 0. Anti-inflammatory foods have a positive number... the higher the number the more they fight inflammation. Inflammatory foods get a negative number. The more negative the number the more inflammatory the food. Use the following chart to see how some common foods rank when it comes to inflammation and let it guide you to reducing your own levels of inflammation.[12] This will help your skin immensely. Don't be afraid to choose foods with a slight negative rating – you can balance them with positive foods – but avoid the ones that are off-the-chart bad like French fries.

Food	Amount	IF Rating
Almonds	¼ cup	+4
Plain bagel	1 bagel	-186
Boiled broccoli	½ cup	+73
Cantaloupe	1 cup	+21
Cheddar cheese	1 ounce	-26
Corn flakes	1 cup	-182
Cottage cheese	½ cup	+9
Whole egg	1 large	-43
French fries, fast food	Medium size	-336
Green beans, cooked	½ cup	+15
Olive oil	1 tablespoon	+73
Pasta shells, cooked	½ cup	-55
Atlantic, farm-raised salmon	3 ounces	-180
Alaskan, wild salmon	3 ounces	+493
Spinach, raw	1 cup	+80

The best supplements for your skin:

Choosing the right foods is an important step to supporting and protecting your skin, but it often isn't enough. Because of modern farming practices, many of the healthiest foods available don't have the level of nutrients they used to. You should take high quality supplements to compensate.

You've already seen how vitamin C works to help your body build the collagen that supports your skin and how vitamin E and CoQ10 help protect your skin from free radical damage. To make sure you are getting enough of these nutrients, supplement with the following each day:

- 1000 mg of vitamin C
- 400 IU of mixed tocopherol vitamin E
- 100 mg of CoQ10

In addition to this, alpha lipoic acid (ALA) will help increase the circulation to your capillaries.[13] Better circulation to your skin helps to nourish and keep it looking youthful. This nutrient is both fat and water soluble allowing it to function throughout the body. It is also known as the "mother antioxidant" for its ability to recharge and restore the effectiveness of other important skin-saving antioxidants, such as vitamin E and vitamin C. Take 100 mg of ALA twice each day.

The best lotions for your skin:

Taking care of your skin from the inside out is important, but it is only half the process. You should also be caring for your skin from the outside in. You can do this by using topical lotions and ointments that are reparative – that help the skin to renew and rejuvenate itself.

Topical lotions that contain vitamin E and vitamin C have a proven protective affect against photodamage.[14] Vitamin C is especially beneficial when used on the skin. In a review of studies, researchers found that the evidence supporting vitamin C as a topical agent to fight photodamage is conclusive. Results showed better collagen production in treated skin, protection from both UV-A and UV-B damage, a reduction in the appearance of age spots, and a reduction in inflammation in the skin.[15]

Topical lotions that contain green tea extracts will also help to protect your skin from photodamage and inflammation. Green tea contains a polyphenol called EGCG. (This stands for epigallocatechin-3 gallate.) In studies, people who applied green tea extract to their skin before going out in the sun experienced less oxidative stress in the skin. The green tea extract also reduced inflammation in the skin, which will help to reduce wrinkles.[16]

Treating Cosmetic Skin Conditions

Implantations – treats crow's-feet and whistle lines around the lips. This is also effective for treating some scars. A number of different substances may be used such as Collagen, Hyaluronic acid and Fat Injections.

Resurfacing – treats fine lines, dryness and blotchiness on the whole face. Several techniques are commonly used such as Alpha hydroxyl acid, Kinerase, Topical retinoic acid, glycolic acid peels, TCA peels, Dermabrasion, Laser resurfacing, nonablative resurfacing and Dr. Sears' "no-peel" peels.

For more information on Dr. Sears' "no-peel" peel, call the office at (561) 784-7852.

Another topical agent that is proven to work is the isoflavone equol. Research shows that right after sun exposure, using a lotion containing the equol reduces inflammation, protects collagen, inhibits photoaging, and helps prevent the development of skin cancers.[17]

There is also the old standby, aloe vera. You are probably familiar with the ability of aloe vera gel to reduce the inflammation related to sunburn. But scientists from the Department of Immunology at the Anderson Cancer Center in Houston have also shown that aloe vera gel protects the skin's immune cells from sun damage.[18] One of the best aloe vera lotions we know of is Lily of the Desert Aloe Vera Gelly. You can find it online or in most health food stores. This product contains only all-natural ingredients, including vitamins A, C and E, all of which have skin saving antioxidant properties.

By using a combination of these topical treatments, you will help your skin stay soft and supple and evenly colored and you will be able to enjoy healthy time in the sun without worrying that you are prematurely aging your skin.

One More Step:

Finally, there is one more step you should take to help prevent skin aging. Your hormone levels affect the health of your skin. Balanced, healthy levels of hormones promote toned, soft skin. As you age, your hormone levels tend to decline and become unbalanced. A visit to your doctor to determine your hormone levels is a good step. If your hormones are out of balance, ask your doctor to prescribe bio-identical hormones tailored to your specific needs. Your doctor can refer you to a compounding pharmacist who can mix a customized prescription for you. If your doctor doesn't know of a compounding pharmacist, you can visit www.iacprx.org to find one in your area.

Put Your Skin Health into Perspective

Sun exposure is only one factor influencing the wrinkling of your skin. A balanced natural diet, a healthy lifestyle, and moderate exposure to sunlight can bring out your true beauty by keeping the skin soft, flexible, and young looking. And remember that moderate sun exposure can actually help you prevent the most deadly type of skin cancer – melanoma.

In future chapters, you'll learn about many other exciting ways the sun can benefit your health and improve your active longevity. You might end up with a few more freckles when you grow to be a wise and grey elder, but you will likely be in far better shape than if you avoid the sun.

In the next chapter, we'll look at the connection between sunshine and the number one cause of death among both men and women in the United States – heart disease. We'll also look at how sunlight helps prevent and decrease inflammation, the real underlying culprit in the modern epidemic of heart disease.

(Endnotes)

1 Hanson KM and Simon JD. (1998) Epidermal trans-urocanic acid and the UV-A induced photoagin of the skin. *Proc Natl Acad Sci USA* 95(18): 10576-78

2 Yamamoto Y. (2001) Role of active oxygen species and antioxidants in photoaging. *J Dermatol Sci* 27 Suppl 1: S1-4

3 Boelsma E, et al. (2001) Nutritional skin care: health effects of micronutrients and fatty acids. *Am J Clin Nutr*; 73(5): 853-64

4 Purba, MB, et al. (2001). Skin wrinkling: Can food make a difference? *J Am Coll Nutr.* 20(1): 71-80.

5 Giacomoni, Paolo. (2005) Ageing, Science, and the Cosmetics Industry. *EMBO Reports*; 6:S45-S48

6 Simopoulos AP. (2006) Evolutionary aspects of diet, the omega 3/omega 6 ratio and genetic variation: nutritional implications of chronic disease. *Biomed Pharmacother;* 60(9): 502-7

7 Scalise, Kathleen. (1997) UC Berkley Press Release: Skin ailments linked to air pollution.

8 Freiman A, et al. (2004) Cutaneos affects of smoking. *J Cutan Med Surg*; 8(6): 415-23

9 Van Wijk EP, et al. (2006) Anatomic characterization of human ultra-weak photo emission in practitioners of transcendental meditation and control subjects. *J altern Complement Med,* 12(1): 31-8

10 *Journal of American College of Nutrition* 2001; 20: 71-80

11 Ulrike H, et al. (2006) Long-term ingestion of high flavanol cocoa provides photoprotection against UV induced erythema and improves skin condition in women. *J Nutr*; 136: 1565-69

12 Reinagel, Monica. *The Inflammation Free Diet Plan.* Lynn Sonberg Book Associates, 2005.

13 Haak E, et al. (2000) Effects of alpha lipoic acid on microcirculation in patients with peripheral diabetic neuropathy, *Exp Clin Endocrinol Diabetes*; 108(3) 168-74

14 Eberlain-Konig B, Ring J. (2005) Relevance of vitamin C and E in cutaneous photoprotection. *J Cosmet Dermatol,* 4(10): 4-9

15 Farris PK. (2005) Topical vitamin C: a useful agent for treating photoaging and other dermatological conditions. *Dermatol Surg*; 31(7pt2): 814-17

16 Katiyar SK, et al. (1999) Polyphenolic antioxidant (-)-epigallocatechin-3-gallate from green tea reduces UVB-induced inflammatory responses and infiltration of leukocytes in human skin. *Photochem Photobiol*; 69(2):148-53.

17 Reeve VE, et al. (2005) Protection against photoaging in the hairlss mouse by the isoflavone equol. *Photochem Photobiol,* 81(6): 1548-53

18 Strickland, FM et al. (1999) Inhibition of UV-induced immune suppression and interleukin-10 production by plant oligosaccharides and polysaccharides. *Photochem Photobiol.* 69(2):141-7.

CHAPTER EIGHT

Prevent the Biggest Killer in the Nation

"Medical men tend to decry and condemn every wholesome thing and practice and laud to the skies every unwholesome thing and practice. To them, only poisons have value in maintaining and restoring health. The normal things of life are suspect. While they repeatedly warn us of the "dangers" of sunbathing, they even more frequently tell us of the virtues of penicillin or arsenic. They are not to be taken seriously, for the reason that their anti-natural approach to all of the problems of life guarantees that they will be on the wrong side of everything."

– Dr. Herbert M. Shelton, 1934

You're enjoying a stroll in the park when sudden pain hits you like a Mack truck out of nowhere. Now you're on your knees, clutching your chest, gasping for air. The frightening scenario of a **heart attack** is all too familiar.

Nearly one million Americans will die from heart disease this year – another record number in a long string of ever increasing record-breaking deaths. Despite our country dutifully buying and swallowing billions of dollars worth of drugs supposed to protect us, heart disease remains the number one killer in the U.S. And in 2004, heart disease, for the first time in history became the number one killer worldwide.

You've heard that narrowing of the arteries causes heart attacks and strokes. Most cardiologists explain this process as a plumbing problem:

Fat and cholesterol build up and narrow arteries.
This prevents oxygen from reaching tissue and it dies.
If the dying tissue is a part of your heart, you have a
heart attack. If it's your brain, you have a stroke.

Yet recent research paints a different picture. Coronary arteries bear only a superficial resemblance to pipes. Closer examination reveals that they're muscles sandwiched between two "structural" layers. When the muscles or the connective tissues become inflamed, heart disease sets in.

This understanding is driving a new model for heart disease prevention. In this chapter, we'll examine the modern causes of this inflammatory phenomenon and how sunlight can prevent and reverse it – dramatically reducing your risk.

Science has made great strides in identifying what causes damage to arteries. Among the biggest culprits are oxidation from a lack of antioxidants in our modern diets and high levels of sugar in the blood from excessive consumption of refined carbohydrates. Excess blood sugar can lead to glycation of proteins, a process that can damage delicate tissues. Both of these conditions are related to recent dietary changes like low vegetable consumption and high consumption of processed starches. A third change is the lack of sunshine.

In short, heart disease is not a disease caused by fat and cholesterol. Instead, **cholesterol is the thing that heart disease acts upon**. The disease is the abnormal amount of oxidation and inflammation. The inflammation occurs within – not on – arterial walls.

Oxidation is normally under control by your specialized "anti-oxidant" system but has been weakened by our modern dietary deficiencies. Inflammation occurs when we expose ourselves to foreign substances alien to our native physiology. Inflammation then leads to a loss of the normal flexibility of our arteries. This is especially critical for the "mechanically stressed" coronary arteries that supply blood to your heart. These factors can also lead to abnormal blood clotting as your body struggles to minimize the damage.

This newer understanding suggests four ways to prevent or reverse this leading killer:

1. Reverse oxidation.
2. Control inflammation.
3. Restore your arteries' flexibility.
4. Reduce abnormal blood clotting.

It may surprise you to know that you can use free and natural sunlight to positively change all four of these heart disease factors.

Sunlight Reduces Your Heart Disease Risk

Facts from many different sources corroborate that people who are exposed to the most sunlight on a regular basis have reduced risks of heart disease. Consider the following:

- Heart attacks are more common during the winter months when sun exposure is at its lowest.[1]

- Night workers who sleep during the daylight hours have twice the rate of heart disease as the general population.

- There are progressively more heart attacks in populations the farther you get from the equator.

- Despite lower oxygen levels there are significantly *fewer* heart disease deaths at higher altitudes where UVB exposure is also highest.

We have known for some time that most long-lived cultures around the world reside at relatively high altitude where sun exposure is the greatest.[2] As early as 1969, researchers Voors and Johnson observed this phenomenon. As altitude increased, death from heart disease decreased. The mortality rates from heart disease in some high-altitude cities are half that of sea-level cities.[3]

African-Americans and others with dark skin are much less reactive to sunshine relative to fair skinned individuals. This may be in part why African Americans have a higher risk of heart disease.

- 20% more deaths from heart disease
- Twice as many suffer from strokes
- 40% have high blood pressure

In addition to these many indirect associations, a number of studies have directly linked heart disease to vitamin D levels. In 1990, Dr. Robert Scragg led a study which showed that heart attacks were twice as common in patients with low vitamin D levels.[4] More than a decade later, Dr. Armin Zitterman performed a study which showed that most of the patients who had experienced heart failure had low levels of vitamin D.[5]

How Can Simple, Free Sunlight Prevent Heart Disease?

Sunshine Lowers Your Blood Sugar

Over time, high blood sugar cause inflammatory "glycation" within your arteries and organ proteins. Glycation is particularly damaging to coronary arteries.[6] This explains why diabetics (people with chronically high blood sugar) have 4.5 times the risk of suffering from heart attack than non-diabetics. Fortunately, you can restore your natural sun exposure to curb this modern danger.

Sunlight literally lowers your blood sugar and increases your sensitivity to insulin. Sunlight helps move glucose out of the blood stream and into your cells and muscles where you burn it for energy. And removing the glucose from your blood stream lowers both inflammation and oxidation in your arteries.

You'll learn in detail how sunlight does this and even fights diabetes in the next chapter.

Sunlight Reduces Inflammation by Boosting Vitamin D

Reducing inflammation is "The Holy Grail" of beating heart disease.

As we have seen, your body uses sunlight to produce vitamin D, in much the same way that plants use the sun to produce food. Like plants that wither away due to lack of sunlight, people slowly die without the vitamin D that sunlight helps them create. Being deficient in vitamin D directly leads to inflammatory diseases such as heart disease.

Vitamin D deficiency is widespread across the nations most afflicted with heart disease. A study of people admitted to a Boston hospital found that 57 percent were deficient in vitamin D. 22 percent were severely deficient.[7]

Vitamin D is a powerful anti-inflammatory. Without it, the inflammation response to oxidation in the arteries goes uncontrolled. What would be harmlessly repaired becomes life threatening.

How can we prove the powerful anti-inflammatory properties of vitamin D? The best test for inflammation inside the blood steam is a blood protein called C-reactive protein, or CRP. This substance is known to be the best "biological marker" for internal inflammation. Doctors use CRP in the blood to measure for total inflammation levels in the body. When the total inflammation is high then there is a corresponding increase in CRP and vice-versa.

- In a study performed at Queen Mary's School of Medicine in London, Vitamin D supplementation lowered three different factors of inflammation, including significantly lowering blood CRP.[8]

- In a Belgian study of critically ill patients with high levels of inflammation, natural vitamin D reduced CRP by more than 25 percent. Another marker for inflammation, IL-6, also fell. These patients only received a small dose of 500 units of vitamin D per day.[9]

Arteries: Relax… Be Happy… With Just a Little Sunshine

If your muscles in your arteries can relax, narrowed arteries aren't as threatening. An artery that can relax and dilate makes it unlikely that ruptured plaque or clots will block the blood flow. The best indicator of your arteries capacity to relax normally is your blood pressure. A lower blood pressure means your arteries relax better.

Before you picked up this book you probably would not have thought of sunlight as a blood pressure lowering therapy, but it's actually one of the best.

We have known for decades that people who live in sunny cli-

Prevent the Biggest Killer in the Nation

mates have, on average, lower blood pressures. Now research is beginning to show us how this occurs.

Dr. Michael Holick has found evidence that vitamin D naturally keeps enzymes that cause blood vessels to constrict in check. In his experiment, Dr. Holick put volunteers with mild hypertension under UV lights for just six minutes, three times a week. This exposure doubled their average vitamin D levels in six weeks. The average blood pressure of the group also dropped significantly with some achieving completely normal blood pressures.[10]

Researchers have known about a link between light and blood pressure at least as early as 1935. In fact, a study published in the American Journal of Physiology showed that UV light reduced blood pressure in hypertensive patients by 60 to 70 percent.

This study also found that a single exposure could sometimes reduce blood pressure immediately. The effect often lasted for two days or more. Multiple exposures on consecutive days reduced blood pressure for a week. [11] Modern studies have also confirmed that the activated form of vitamin D has the ability to reduce blood pressure.[12]

Large population studies also support the beneficial effect of sunshine on arteries:

- Blood pressure is lower at latitudes closer to the equator.
- Blood pressure is lower at higher altitudes.
- Blood pressure is lower in the summer months.
- Blood pressure is higher in African Americans, in the aged, and in the obese. (These are all vitamin D deficient populations.)
- People from cultures that live predominantly outside have almost no high blood pressure.

- The Maryland Heart Association discovered that people living in nudists colonies have high blood pressure at only half the national average. [13]

Sunlight Prevents Abnormal Blood Clotting

We have known that heart attacks decrease in the summer and increase in the winter. For years, researchers believed this might be due to changes in temperatures themselves. Recently evidence suggests a more plausible mechanism. A small but growing amount of research shows that vitamin D may protect against heart disease by decreasing the risk of clot formation.[14]

The beneficial effect of sunshine on blood clotting also shows up among surgical patients. 10 percent of post-surgery patients who don't get any sunlight exposure experience excess blood clotting. In sharp contrast, in one study, patients treated with sun exposure prior to or directly after surgery did not have a single clotting complication.[15]

Studies among mice also help us understand the relationship between sunshine and blood clotting. Recently, scientists demonstrated that the photosynthesis of vitamin D helps activate genes that prevent excess blood clotting. Without vitamin D, these genes remain dormant and blood clotting goes uncontrolled.[16]

These four mechanisms alone could have a powerful beneficial effect on the heart disease risks of millions of people around the world.

Action of Vitamin D:	Protects Heart By:
Increases insulin sensitivity	Reduces blood sugar, decreasing risk of glycation of arteries.

Reduces inflammation	Breaks the cycle of inflammation cascade in the arteries.
Lowers blood pressure	Helps endothelial cells function properly, allowing arteries to relax.
Activates genes that prevent excessive blood clotting	Reduce the number of clots that could trigger heart attack.

Sunshine May Lower Your Cholesterol

If you receive proper sun exposure, you're also likely to have lower cholesterol levels. The explanation for this is really quite simple:

There's a rich supply of cholesterol stored in your skin. When exposed to ultraviolet light, your body converts this cholesterol to vitamin D.[17] As this cholesterol is depleted from the skin, it is replenished by cholesterol from the blood. This explains why people experience a rapid and sharp decrease in blood cholesterol when exposed to sunlight.[18]

The link between sun exposure and lower cholesterol is clear:

- Cholesterol measurements are higher at latitudes further from the equator[19]

- Cholesterol is higher at lower altitudes[20]

- Cholesterol is higher in the winter[21]

- The seasonal variations in cholesterol have been well studied and can not be explained by seasonal dietary changes.[22]

Without enough sun exposure, concentrations of cholesterol in the blood begin to rise. Consider the results of a few more studies which show the correlation between sun exposure and cholesterol levels.

- **Two-hour exposure to sunlight dropped cholesterol levels** – cholesterol levels were taken before exposure to sunlight. 97 percent of the patients experienced a reduction in cholesterol after sun exposure. The average drop was 15 percent after only one two-hour exposure, and more than 80 percent of the subjects maintained this reduction for 24 hours. [23]

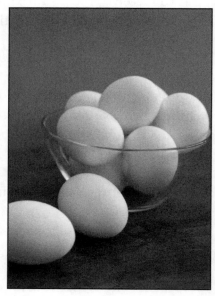

- **Light makes lower-cholesterol eggs** – Chickens raised under full-spectrum lights produce eggs with 25% lower cholesterol content.[24]

- **Four days of sun exposure dropped cholesterol and triglycerides** – A powerful case study by Dr. Zane Kime, MD reports of a female patient whose cholesterol was 333 ml/dl and triglycerides were 299 mg/dl. After four days of sun exposure, with no changes in diet or exercise, the woman's cholesterol and triglycerides had dropped to 221 and 197 mg/dl respectively – more than a 100-point drop in both indexes.

Prevent the Biggest Killer in the Nation

Take these Steps to Sidestep
Our Epidemic of Heart Disease

Cardiologists are quick to prescribe medicine and tell you to watch what you eat when it comes to preventing heart disease, but probably fewer than two in a hundred would think to check your vitamin D levels. But the evidence is clear. Your vitamin D status is extremely important when it comes to your risk of coronary heart disease, heart attack and stroke.

Here are some measures you can take today to lower your risk of heart disease naturally:

- Make sure you have an adequate supply of vitamin D by exposing at least 80 percent of your body to the sun every other day. Review chapter 3 for guidelines to supplement with vitamin D in the winter months.

- Get back your native antioxidants. Eat plenty of vegetables and avoid starches. Build your meals around high quality, lean protein and brightly colored veggies.

- Get a double dose of heart health by exercising outdoors. You'll boost your physical activity and your vitamin D production at the same time. Swimming is a great summer exercise you should enjoy, but avoid chlorination when possible. Salt water swimming is best. A simple walk in the sun is still a great way to build health and help prevent heart disease. You'll find a specific exercise program in chapter 11.

- Finally, if you smoke, quit.

(Endnotes)

1 Pell, JP, Cobbe, SM. (1999). Seasonal variations in coronary heart disease. *Q J Med*. 92(12): 689-96.

2 Leaf, A. (1973). Getting old. *Sci Am*. 229(3):44-52.

3 Voors AW, Johnson WD. (1979). Altitude and arteriosclerotic heart disease mortality in white residents of 99 of the 100 largest cities in the United States. *J Chronic Dis*. 32(1-2):157-62.

4 Scragg R, et al. Myocardial infarction is inversely associated with plasma 25-hydroxyvitamin D3 levels: a community-based study. Int J Epidemiol. 1990 Sep;19(3):559-63

5 Zitterman A, et al. Patients with congestive heart failure (CHF) usually have very low levels of vitamin D. J Am Coll Cardiol. 2003 Jan 1;41(1):105-12.

6 The process of glycation accelerates when the body is insensitive to insulin and glucose remains in the bloodstream and begins to react with amino acids. The product of this reaction is an artery scarring molecule known as an AGE product. Aptly named, this stands for advanced glycated end-product. When formed, they can damage the mechanically stressed coronary arteries and lead to heart disease.

7 "Vitamin D deficiency appears common in hospital patients," Massachusetts General Hospital. March 18, 1998.

8 Timms PM, et al. (2002). Circulating MMP9, vitamin D and variation in the TIMP-1 response with VDR genotype: mechanisms for inflammatory damage in chronic disorders? QJM. 95(12):787-96.

9 Van den Berghe, G. (2003). Bone turnover in prolonged critical illness: effect of vitamin D. *J Clin Endocrinol Metab*. 88(10):4623-32.

10 Krause R, Holick MF, et al. "Ultraviolet B and blood pressure," *Lancet* 1998; 352(9129): 709-10

11 Johnson, JR, et al. (1935). The effect of carbon arc radiation on blood pressure and cardiac output. *American Journal of Physiology*. 114:594.

Prevent the Biggest Killer in the Nation

12 Lind L, et al. (1988). Reduction of blood pressure by treatment with alpha-calcidol. A double-blind, placebo-controlled study in subjects with impaired glucose tolerance. *Acta Med Scand.* 223(3):211-7.

13 Rostand, SG. (1997). Ultraviolet light may contribute to geographic and racial blood pressure differences. *Hypertension.* 30(2 pt 1): 150-6.

Fiori, G, et al. (2000). Relationships between blood pressure, anthropometric characteristics and blood lipids in high- and low-altitude populations from Central Asia. *Ann Hum Biol.* 27(1): 19-28.

Komaroff, AL. (2005). By the way, doctor. My systolic blood pressure is 40 points higher in winter than in the summer (160-180 versus 120-140 mm Hg). Do the seasons affect blood pressure. *Harv Health Lett.* 30(11):8.

14 Scragg, R. (1981). Seasonality of cardiovascular disease mortality and the possible protective effect of ultra-violet radiation. *Int J Epidemiol.* 10(4):337-41.

15 McDonagh, EW. Photoluminescence: UV lght irradiation in the laboratory. The Healing Power of Light.
http://www.lightparty.com/Health/HealingLight.html

16 Ken-ichi, A. (2004). Disruption of Nuclear Vitamin D Receptor Gene Causes Enhanced Thrombogenicity in Mice. *J Biol Chem.* 279(34): 35798-802.

17 Rauschkolb EW, et al. (1971). Effects of Ultraviolet Light on Skin Lipid Metabolism. *J Invest Derm.* 56:387.

18 Altschul, R. (1955). Ultraviolet Irradiation and Cholesterol Metabolism. *Arch Phys Med.* 36:394.

19 Grimes, DS, et al. (1996). Sunlight, cholesterol and coronary heart disease. *QJM.* 89(8):579-89.

20 Baibas, N. (2005). Residence in mountainous compared with lowland areas in relation to total and coronary mortality. *J Epidemiol Community Health.* 59(4):274-8.

21 Gordon, DJ. (1988). Cyclic seasonal variation in plasma lipid and lipoprotein levels: the Lipid Research Clinics Coronary Primary Prevention Trial Placebo Group. *J Clin Epidemiol.* 41(7):679-89.

22 Bluher, M. (2001). <u>Influence of dietary intake and physical activity on annual rhythm of human blood cholesterol concentrations.</u> *Chronobiol Int.* 18(3):541-57.

23 Altschul R, Herman, IH. (1953). Ultraviolet irradiation and Cholesterol metabolism: Seventh Annual meeting of the American Society for the Study of Arteriosclerosis. *Circulation.* 8:438.

24 Liberman, J. (1991). *Light: Medicine of the Future.* Rochester, VT: Bear & Company. p. 59

CHAPTER NINE

Beat This Modern Day Plague

*"The doctor of the future will interest his patients
in the care of the human frame, in diet, and in
the cause and prevention of disease."*

– Thomas A. Edison

A dult diabetes is our modern day plague. An estimated 20.8 million people in the U.S. have this kind of diabetes – 7 percent of the population and rapidly climbing. This condition used to be seen only infrequently and in the elderly. Now we see it striking more and more and younger and younger people.

Modern medicine uses an arsenal of drugs to control and treat the symptoms, but they insist that the disease has no cure. And, the drugs they use to treat the symptoms risk serious side effects–including, paradoxically, obesity.

Yet if you appreciate how modern changes to your environment have caused our current epidemic, natural solutions follow. These natural solutions are safe and effective and have already reversed diabetes in thousands of patients.

Recent studies prove that once again, good old sunshine, coupled with reversing modern worsening of several key nutrient choices, can play an important role in warding off or even curing existing diabetes.

Understanding Diabetes Types

Two different diseases use the term sugar diabetes. Early doctors named them the same because they both result in high blood sugars. This was before we knew that they have two unrelated causes.

Type 1 diabetes is also known as childhood diabetes. It is a genetic disease that results from a mutation to the gene that produces insulin. A small and relatively constant percentage of children are born with this mutation and develop the disease early in life. Since they can't make insulin effectively, injecting insulin, although imperfect and inconvenient is an effective treatment.

In some cases, Type 1 diabetes has been shown to be related to vitamin D deficiency of the pregnant mother. Also, a very large Finnish study showed that supplementation in infants (less than one year of age) and children with 2,000 IU of vitamin D per day reduced the incidence of type 1 diabetes by around 80%. Studies have also shown that supplementation with cod liver oil can produce a similar reduction in the incidence of type 1 diabetes.

People with **type 2 diabetes** or adult onset diabetes do not have a genetic mutation which causes abnormal insulin function. Those who develop this disease are born with normal insulin. We can also remind ourselves of the cause of most adult diabetes with the term "environmental diabetes." It is our modern diet that has caused the rise of adult onset diabetes. Too much starch and sugar trigger the pancreas to overproduce insulin until, just like "crying wolf", the body eventually becomes resistant to the effects of insulin causing blood sugar to climb.

Why Has Diabetes Gone Epidemic?

Insulin's main role is to escort glucose, or blood sugar, and many other nutrients out of the bloodstream and into the muscle cells where you burn it for fuel. Your cells need this to stay alive and energized. However, when the body produces too much insulin for too long it no longer does its job well.

Normal insulin production in a healthy individual is about 31 units per day. Yet a person with adult diabetes can average 114 units per day![1] Similar to people who consume excess alcohol and develop a resistance to it, people with chronically high insulin levels become resistant.

When cells become resistant to insulin, excess blood glucose remains in the bloodstream eventually damaging your cells. You begin to feel tired, grumpy, foggy, and weak. You become pre-diabetic, and if left unchecked, this vicious cycle of insulin resistance will lead to diabetes.

The insulin and glucose overload leads to malnutrition, obesity, hypertension, vision loss, heart disease, diabetes and even cancer. In women, it can cause polycystic ovarian syndrome, which leads to infertility. In men, it can lead to erectile dysfunction. In both men and women, the aging process accelerates, making you look and feel older.

Regain Your Ancestral Blood Sugar Stabilizer

Several factors have caused our modern epidemic of insulin resistance. You will learn how to reverse them in the next section of this chapter. But first, one you're not likely to hear about from your doctor – correct your deficiency of "vitamin sunshine".

In 1998, Professor Boucher of Royal London Hospital Medical & Dental School proposed that vitamin D deficiency caused by deficient sun exposure is a primary factor in insulin resistance. We know that the beta cells in your pancreas that make insulin have specific receptors for vitamin D. And, there are many statistical associations supporting the conclusion that vitamin D is critical for normal insulin metabolism – independent of other nutritional factors.

A study published in the *American Journal of Clinical Nutrition* showed that among those with lower than normal vitamin D levels, 30 percent had one or more symptoms of insulin resistance, compared with only 11 percent of those with normal vitamin D levels.[2]

Similarly, Australian researchers found that low vitamin D levels predispose people to adult diabetes. They discovered that as vitamin D levels decreased, blood sugar and insulin levels increased.[3] This increase is what eventually leads to insulin resistance. A pre-diabetic condition follows and sometimes diabetes. The researchers concluded that the epidemic of diabetes is in part due to the modern day sun avoidance that leads to vitamin D deficiency.

A popular American study known as The Nurses Health Study shows this same correlation. Women who received 800 units of vitamin D a day reduced their risk of developing diabetes by a whopping one-third compared to women who were given only 400 units of vitamin D.[4]

Those most at risk for vitamin D deficiency are also at risk for diabetes. These populations share an increased risk for both D deficiency and diabetes.

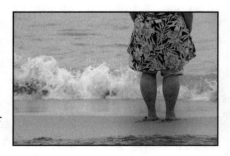

- Those who live in sun-deprived areas of the globe
- The elderly
- The obese
- Those who regularly wear clothing that covers most of their skin

Beat This Modern Day Plague

- Those who live and work indoors
- Those who regularly use chemical sunscreen

You Can Reverse Diabetes with Sunlight

To reverse adult diabetes, you have to make your body sensitive to insulin again. Sunlight and vitamin D help improve insulin sensitivity, helping to restore metabolic balance. Sunlight and vitamin D are more effective than the drug therapy that so many doctors choose as your first (and only) option. Let's take a look…

In the *American Journal of Clinical Nutrition*, Ken C. Chiu and colleagues found that increasing a person's blood concentration of vitamin D from 25 nmol/l to about 75 nmol/l would improve insulin sensitivity by 60 percent. This is a much greater improvement than the current best anti-diabetic drug, metformin, which only gives about a 13 percent improvement in insulin sensitivity.[5]

Other studies produced similar results. In one study using 1,332 IU of vitamin D per day for only 30 days improved insulin sensitivity by 21 percent in 10 women with adult diabetes.[6]

How Sunlight Reduces the Main Risk Factors of Diabetes		
Condition	**Link to diabetes**	**How sunlight helps**
Insulin resistance	Body tries to make more insulin, eventually tiring out the cells that make insulin	Increases the vitamin D necessary for adequate insulin secretion

High blood sugar	Sugar remains in the blood instead of going to the cells in muscles, fat, kidneys and other organs	Increases glycogen production, the form in which blood sugar is stored in the muscles
Low vitamin D levels	Blood sugar increases as vitamin D levels decrease	Vitamin D from sunlight helps protect production of insulin in the pancreas

One explanation for the insulin sensitizing effect of sunlight is that it increases the production of an **enzyme known as glycogen synthetase**. This enzyme causes muscle tissues to produce more glycogen from blood glucose. Because glycogen production lowers blood sugar, it puts less demand on the pancreas to produce insulin. Lower insulin allows cells to recover from insulin resistance.

Glycogen storage also controls appetite. Controlling your appetite prevents overeating and subsequent high blood sugar. This is yet another way to decrease insulin production and lower insulin resistance.

Sunshine allows you to produce and store more glycogen in your muscles. Your body derives energy from stored glycogen between meals. If glycogen storage is low then hunger sets in quickly. This is one reason diabetics may have increased appetite – they have very little glycogen storage. Healthy amounts of glycogen in your muscles serve as a "sugar reserve system."

Beat This Modern Day Plague

A vitamin D deficiency or lack of sun exposure can also lead to hyperparathyroidism. Hyperparathyroidism means an excess production of parathyroid hormone (PTH). Too much PTH causes excessive levels of calcium to become stored within fat and muscle cells. The excess calcium can block the cell's ability to respond to the insulin inducing insulin resistance.[7]

Sensitize Your Insulin with the Sunshine Vitamin

Now is a good time to optimize your vitamin D with sun exposure. Not only will doing this increase your general health and well-being, but it can help protect you from diabetes by:

- Lowering blood sugar
- Restoring insulin sensitivity
- Increasing the production of glycogen
- Curbing your appetite
- And, preventing hyperparathyroidism.

You can prevent diabetes. Ask your doctor to give you a simple blood test to check your vitamin D levels. (See chapter 3 for more information on getting tested.) Then use a combination of sunlight, vitamin D supplementation, and dietary sources to obtain optimal levels.

Certain populations such as the obese, elderly and African-Americans can't photosynthesize vitamin D as well. Supplementation with vitamin D rich cod liver oil is vital for optimal health among these groups. (See chapter 4 for specific guidelines on supplementing with vitamin D.)

Increasing your vitamin D is vital, but it should not be your only step to prevent insulin resistance. Below is a guide for things you can do to protect yourself from type 2 diabetes.

Putting It All Together: Steps to Prevent Diabetes

Step 1: Reverse the dietary changes causing the epidemic of diabetes. A poor diet is the main cause of diabetes. You can reverse three simple dietary changes that will almost guarantee you won't get diabetes.

- First, reduce your intake of anything made from grains or potatoes. Grain products include breads, cereals and pastas. And remember, corn is a grain.

  These contain a lot of starch, which feeds chronically high glucose levels. Start changing the amount of grain in your diet slowly. Eliminate grains at breakfast, then at lunch, and finally at snacks and dinner until you use them only sparingly.

- Second, don't buy any foods that contain high fructose corn syrup. This high calorie sweetener is worse than pure sugar. This man-made product plays a trick on your system that regulates satiation. No matter how much you eat you don't feel full. Too much food and soft drinks with high fructose corn syrup and you'll be fat, tired **and** diabetic.

- Finally, eliminate *trans* fats from your diet. These man-made fats are bad for you in a lot of ways. They are even worse for diabetics. You will find them in processed vegetable oils. Simply don't buy anything with the word "hydrogenated" anywhere on the label.

Step 2: Exercise. We all know that exercise is important, but we often don't realize what exercise is best. To prevent diabetes, interval training is best – short bursts of high intensity exercise spaced between intervals of more relaxed activity. This kind of exercise promotes glycogen storage and fat burning.

Be sure to work your larger muscles of your legs and back. Biking, dance, or swimming are all good ways to exercise these muscles. When you work these muscles, you burn off large amounts of your glycogen stores. The body then pulls excess glucose from the blood stream to replenish those stores.

Step 3: Schedule time every day to go out in the sun. If your time is limited, then try to go out around mid-day. Don't put on sunscreen or sunglasses. Just bask in the sun's glow for 15 or 20 minutes. It's even better if you can do this more than once in a day.

One More Natural Tip...

In a recent study, even a small daily dose of cinnamon reduced fasting blood sugar levels by up to 29 percent.[8] This same study also found that cinnamon reduced triglyceride and cholesterol levels.

Use a quarter of teaspoon of cinnamon every day. Try it on applesauce or in yogurt. Cinnamon tea is also good.

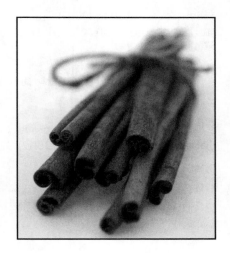

(Endnotes)

1 Whitaker, J. (2001). *Reversing Diabetes: Reduce or Even Eliminate Your Dependence on Insulin or Oral Drugs.* New York: Warner Books, Inc.

2 Gaby, A. (2004). Prevent diabetes and insulin resistance with vitamin D. Health Notes Newswire. http://www.pccnaturalmarkets.com/health/Newswire/Back_issues/newswire_2004_06_17_2.htm

3 Need, AG, et al. (2005). Relationship between fasting serum glucose, age, body mass index and serum 25 hydroxyvitamin D in postmenopausal women. *Clin Endocrinol (Oxf)*. 62(6):738-41.

4 Pittas, AG, et al. "Vitamin D and calcium intake in relation to type 2 diabetes in women," *Diabetes Care* 2006; 29: 650-56

5 Chiu, KC, et al. (2004). Hypovitaminosis D is associated with insulin resistance and beta cell dysfunction. *Am J Clin Nutr*. 79(5):820-5.

6 Borissova, AM, et al. (2003). The effect of vitamin D3 on insulin secretion and peripheral insulin sensitivity in type 2 diabetic patients. *Int J Clin Pract*. 57(4):258-61.

7 McCarty, MF. (2004). Vitamin D, parathyroid hormone, and insulin sensitivity. *Am J Clin Nutr*. 80(5):1451-2.

8 Khan A, et al. "Cinnamon improves glucose and lipids of people with type 2 diabetes," *Diabetes Care* 2003; 26(12): 3215-18

CHAPTER TEN

Become a Disease-Fighting Dynamo

"When a small amount of blood is treated through photoluminescence, an astounding thing happens. Through some mechanism that is not completely understood, the body's defenses are organized rapidly to destroy all invading organisms, whether viral, fungal, or bacterial. The immune system comes to life and rapidly brings the body back to a state of balance."[1]

– William Campbell Douglas II

You don't think about it in your daily routine but you live in a state of continuous biological warfare. Microbial invaders are testing your defenses as your read this. Viruses, bacteria, fungi and parasites use their millions of years of evolution-earned tricks to try and gain the upper hand in the battle – and eat you alive.

The reason you don't usually notice this life-and-death struggle is that you have one of the greatest wonders in all of biology dutifully and automatically wining this battle for you – your immune system. Take it away and the attacking hordes win, have you for lunch, and you die a most unpleasant death within days.

So with this wondrous defense system, why do some people get sick more than others? And why, throughout most of the populated world, do people get sick more often in winter? Something about the winter must compromise our immune defense.

As you'll soon see, our native sun, from which we have all but divorced ourselves, forms a critical element in a strong immune defense. Sunlight not only ramps up your defenses, but it also fine tunes your response to make fewer mistakes. You'll see how important this is because mistakes of your immune system, like "friendly fire" in war, can sometimes do as much damage to your health as the enemy.

The following chart shows how profoundly and directly sunshine impacts the cells of your immune system.

Sunlight Stimulates Cells of Your Immune System	
Sunlight	**Your Immune System**
Increases the number of white blood cells in the human body	These white blood cells play a leading role in defending your body against bacteria, viruses, parasites and fungi.
Increases lymphocytes responsible for fighting disease.	Lymphocytes produce antibodies and interferon which stop the reproduction of viruses and growth of cancers.
Increases neutrophils	A specific kind of white blood cell, neutorphils form a front line of defense against microbes, especially bacteria.
Vitamin D regulates the immune system.	It can make it stronger, or turn off your immune response when it is out of control (autoimmune illness)
Increases the oxygen content in the cells	More oxygen causes cancer cells to slow or stop their growth and stimulates your immune cells.

Become a Disease-Fighting Dynamo

The Sun Moderates Immunity Too

Your immune system also uses cells called macrophages to fight disease. They work like little "pac men" in your cells. Macrophages ingest any invading, unwanted substances. When you have an infection, macrophages help to fight it. But if they get over-stimulated, they begin to destroy healthy tissue as well.

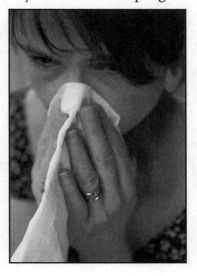

German researchers Laura Helming and Andreas Lengeling recently found that vitamin D helps regulate macrophages. It holds their cytokine production back, so they don't spiral out of control and damage their owner along with the invaders.[2]

This helps to explain the frequency of autoimmune illness in vitamin D deficient patients. Without enough activated vitamin D, there is nothing to tell the macrophages "enough already!"

Sunlight Helps Relieve Autoimmune Diseases

More than 80 conditions fall into the category of autoimmune diseases. With these diseases, your body's own immune system becomes confused. It goes into overdrive and begins attacking your own tissue, ultimately harming you.

Autoimmune diseases can affect different parts of the body. There are conditions that attack the endocrine system, gastrointestinal system, skin, muscles, or the neuromuscular system. Some syndromes affect more than one organ or system.

Vitamin D regulates immune function. We know that vitamin D suppresses autoimmunity and vitamin D deficiency increases the severity of autoimmune illnesses. But how vitamin D helps regulate the immune system is just now coming to light.[3]

Scientists are now looking at creating vitamin D analogs to use in immunosuppressive therapies.[4] But if you have an autoimmune disorder, a sensible strategy should include moderate sun exposure.

Sunlight shows promise in treating and preventing autoimmune disorders like rheumatoid arthritis and multiple sclerosis.

Protect Yourself from Pain and Inflammation

Arthritis is a very common and growing problem. In fact, an estimated 43 million adult Americans suffer pain from arthritis. The Centers for Disease Control estimates that by 2020 sixty million adults will be afflicted with arthritis.[5]

One of the most devastating types of arthritis is rheumatoid arthritis or RA. RA is an autoimmune disease. That means that a mistake of the immune system causes it to attack the cells of the body instead of the microbial enemy. In rheumatoid arthritis, white blood cells attack the lining of the joints causing inflammation. The white blood cells may eventually attack the cartilage, as well. This leads to pain and joint damage.

It may take years to cause a visible deformity of the joint, but we now know that bone and cartilage damage begins in the first couple of years after rheumatoid arthritis sets in, making early diagnosis and treatment paramount.

Sunlight Health Research Center, recently reported a clinical trial where vitamin D helped reduce the activity of rheumatoid arthritis. Vitamin D "therapy showed a positive effect on disease activity in 89 percent of the patients (45 percent with complete remission and 45 percent with a satisfactory effect). Only two patients (11 percent) showed no improvement, but no new symptoms occurred."[6]

Arthritis & Rheumatism reported that supplementing with at least 400 IU of vitamin D each day reduces the risk of rheumatoid arthritis by 34 percent. Remember, 400 IU is barely enough to just prevent bone loss. Now imagine the risk reduction that could result from receiving optimal levels of vitamin D each day. A 1996 study also showed that arthritis progressed more rapidly in those with low vitamin D intake.[7] And lastly, an Iowa Women's Health Study of nearly 30,000 women in their 50s and 60s found that rheumatoid arthritis went down as dietary vitamin D increased.

If you have RA, get your vitamin D levels tested. If your levels are low follow the recommendations in this book to aggressively boost your vitamin D to a blood level of 50. With proper supplementation, you can reduce your risk, slow the progression of the disease and even relieve symptoms.

Prevent a Lifelong Degenerative Condition

As many as 2.5 million people worldwide have Multiple Sclerosis. About 250,000 people in the U.S. have this potentially devastating disease. MS is a degenerative disease that disrupts communication between the brain and other parts of the body.

MS is an autoimmune disease that affects the central nervous system (CNS). It causes the body's immune system to attack its own tissues – in this case, the myelin sheath that insulates the nerves. It is still not fully understood what causes these neurological "short circuits." Since there is no cure for MS, and the medicine used to treat it often comes with serious side effects, prevention is key.

A recent study performed by Kassandra L. Munger of the Harvard School of Public Health in Boston showed evidence of a protective effect of vitamin D against MS. In two studies of almost 200,000 nurses, those women who get at least 400 IU of vitamin D per day showed 40 percent less risk of developing MS compared with those getting less vitamin D.

This corresponds with numerous population studies which show that the incidence and severity of MS is much higher in the geographic regions that receive less sunlight.

Here is more of what we know about the connection between vitamin D levels and multiple sclerosis:

1. **Low vitamin D intake raises your risk** – There is a lot of evidence to show that low vitamin D intake is a key risk factor for MS. A study by Harvard University shows that supplementing with 400 IU per day of vitamin D cut the risk of MS by 40 percent.[8] Again, imagine what optimal levels could do.

2. **Vitamin D decreases the intensity of the autoimmune response** – Vitamin D helps the immune system distinguish body tissues from foreign material. In MS the body mistakes the tissues that insulate nerves as foreign and works to destroy it. Vitamin D decreases the intensity of the autoimmune response and reduces the severity of symptoms.

3. **Vitamin D produces anti-inflammatory effects** – Inflammation is a hallmark of MS. A natural "immuno-regulator," vitamin D produces anti-inflammatory effects.

4. **Sunlight exposure reduces risk** – Studies show that people who were exposed to a lot of sunlight in their childhood are less likely to get the disease. Frequent sunburns in childhood are actually associated with reduced risk of multiple sclerosis

Become a Disease-Fighting Dynamo

later in life.[9] Obviously it is not the sunburns, but the sun exposure.

5. **Occupation and residential sun exposure reduces risk** – Researchers in Maryland studied all deaths from MS over a 10 year period in 24 states. They found that people who get sun exposure as part of their job had lower mortality from MS. Higher degrees of sun exposure reduced the incidence of death by as much as 76 percent.[10]

Prevent Parkinson's Disease with Vitamin D

Korean researchers discovered that vitamin D functions like a natural anti-inflammatory agent that can help prevent Parkinson's disease. The study involved 85 Parkinson's patients and a control group of 200 healthy patients. The study showed that variations or mutations in a vitamin D receptor gene made the Parkinson's patients more susceptible to the disease.[11]

Benefit Every Day from a Healthier Immune Defense

We've come a long way in fighting infectious disease over the past 150 years. Improvements in sanitation, nutrition, and living conditions have all helped put an end to disease. Yet research proves that we should not cut our ties to sunshine and the many ways it boosts our defense to infectious diseases:

1. **Flu and cancer causing viruses** – UV light destroys the flu virus outside the body. In 1976, Heding found that UV light could destroy cancer-causing viruses.[12]

2. **Chronic viral infections in the blood** – Sunlight passes through the outer layers of the skin. It irradiates the blood in the capillaries, helping to kill chronic viral infections.

3. **Decontaminating blood used for transfusions** – New technologies can decontaminate blood using UV light. Using the photosensitive chemical Photofrin combined with UV radiation, researchers have been able to kill 100 percent of the viruses causing AIDS, cold sores, and other illnesses without damaging healthy blood cells.[13]

4. **Bacteria on us and around us** – Sun exposure increases your resistance to illness. Not only do the UV rays kill germs on the surface of your skin, but sun exposure also causes the oils within the skin to have their own bactericidal effect.

Building your immune system pays big benefits in overall health. With a stronger immune system, you reduce your chances of getting a cold or the flu. You also have the ability to fight off infectious diseases and any other pathogens.

Vitamin D deficiency linked to post-Winter flu outbreaks?

A team of researchers are gathering data in an attempt to determine why flu outbreaks hit the Northern hemisphere during winter months and tend to peak between December and March, and a new theory suggest it may be a lack of sunshine-produced vitamin D.

Theories about a chill causing the diseases's prevalence is upended by evidence from tropical locations, where flu remains common and follows a similar seasonal patter to its cold-climate counterpart. The grouping theory is debunked by the fact that certain groups of people are stuck in small spaces together year round, with no grater likelihood of contracting flu than anyone else.

The tropical evidence that upsets the chill theory does not prelude the vitamin D theory, as some researchers point out, as studies show that vitamin D deficiencies have even been recorded in equatorial locations. Additionally, a 2003 analysis of flu cases found they were greatest during the rainy season, when there is a significant cloud cover and reduced sun exposure.

Become a Disease-Fighting Dynamo

Reinforce Sunlight's Immune Effectiveness

Other research suggests that vitamin D has stronger immune boosting and cancer fighting effects when it is in the presence of antioxidants.[14]

To strengthen you immunity, especially in winter, take action to make sure you are getting enough antioxidants. The most potent antioxidants are vitamins E and C, beta carotene, and coenzyme Q10. Herbs and spices like rosemary and curcumin are also loaded with antioxidants.

Start by checking your multivitamin. You want to get 1000 mg of vitamin C, 400 IU of mixed tocopherol vitamin E, and 100 mg of CoQ10. Beta carotene and other carotenoids help your body to create vitamin A. You want to get enough mixed carotenoids for 25,000 IU of vitamin A activity.

If your multivitamin doesn't contain these doses, you'll want to add in other supplements to give your antioxidants a boost.

Of course, the best way to get your antioxidants is through food. Brightly colored fruits and vegetables are good sources of vitamins C and beta carotene. Grass-fed beef and fish are good sources of vitamin E and Coenzyme Q10.

Finally, make a commitment to use more fresh herbs and spices in your cooking. Herbs and spices are dense in antioxidants and they add variety and flavor.

(Endnotes)

1 Douglass, WC. (2003). *Into the Light: Tomorrow's Medicine Today*. Panama City, Panama: Rhino Publishing. p. 11.

2 Helming L, et al. "1alpha,25-Dihydroxyvitamin D3 is a potent suppressor of interferon gamma-mediated macrophage activation," *Blood* 2005; 106(13): 4351-58

3 Cantorna, MT. (2000). Vitamin D and autoimmunity: is vitamin D status an environmental factor affecting autoimmune disease prevalence? *Proc.Soc.Exp. Biol.Med.* 223:230-3.

4 Muller, K, Bendtzen, K. (1996). 1,25-Dihydroxyvitamin D3 as a natural regulator of human immune functions. *J Investig Dermatol Symp Proc.* 1(1):68-71.

5 "Arthritis," The Mayday Pain Project.

6 Clin. Exp. Rheumatol. 1999 (17): pp. 453-456

7 McAlindon, TE, et al. (1996). Relation of dietary intake and serum levels of vitamin D to progression of osteoarthritis of the knee among participants in the Framingham Study. *Ann Intern Med.* 125(5):353-9.

8 Munger KL, et al. "Vitamin D intake and incidence of multiple sclerosis," *Neurology* 2004; 62(1): 60-5

9 van der Mei, IA, et al. (2003). Past exposure to sun, skin phenotype, and risk of multiple sclerosis: case-control study. BMJ. 327(7410):316.

10 Freedmana, DM, et al. (2000). Mortality from multiple scleroris and exposure to residential and occupational solar radiationi: a case-control study based on death certificates. *Occup Environ Med.* 57:418-421.

11 Kim, JS, et al. (2005). Association of vitamin D receptor gene polymorphism and Parkinson 's disease in Koreans. *Journal of Korean Medical Science.* 20(3):495-98.

12 Kime, ZR. (1980). *Sunlight.* Penryn, CA: World Health Publications. p. 164.

13 Liberman, J. (1991). *Light: Medicine of the Future.* Rochester, VT: Bear & Company. p. 115.

14 Danilenko, M, Studzinski GP. "Enhancement by other compounds of the anti-cancer activity of vitamin D(3) and its analogs," *Exp Cell Res* 2004; 298(2): 339-58.

CHAPTER ELEVEN

Solar Powered Fitness

"There is muscular energy in sunlight corresponding to the spiritual energy of wind."

– Annie Dillard

Sunlight and your good health go hand in hand. Not only does your native sun help prevent life-threatening diseases like cancer, heart disease, and diabetes; it also has an incredibly broad array of positive effects on your health, strength, physical performance and quality of life.

When you get regular exposure to sunlight, you enjoy a higher immunity to infection, stronger bones, lower risk of arthritis, greater neurological and mental health, better eyesight and quicker recovery from injury, illness, and pain. You'll also enjoy better fitness, react better to stress, think sharper and work better.

You can take advantage of all of these health improvements with simple adjustments to your daily routine. And, best of all, they're all free.

Let's take a closer look at some of these diverse health benefits.

Want to get more for the same amount of time? You can supercharge your exercise routine. Simply move your favorite exercise outdoors. Use any of the many ways to incorporate sunshine into your exercise plan and you'll notice greater energy, stamina, muscular development and overall fitness!

Sunlight Makes Your Body Stronger

Sunlight literally boosts your metabolism much like exercise does. It boosts balance, strength and muscle mass. Dozens of studies show that sunlight improves athletic performance. Sunshine helps you lose weight, it protects your teeth from cavities, and it lowers your chances of getting cataracts as you age.

Peak Your Athletic Performance

Have you ever noticed most world records in many sporting events are broken in the summer? This is true.

This is because vitamin D is produced in the body when exposed to the sun. So events such as swimming, track, baseball, football and soccer are all outdoors and the players are exposed to sunlight.

The active form of vitamin D is a steroid in the same way that testosterone is a steroid and vitamin D is a hormone in the same way that growth hormone is a hormone. That is, both vitamin D and testosterone regulate your genome, the stuff of life. While testosterone is a sex hormone, vitamin D is a multiple function steroid hormone.

Certainly steroids can improve athletic performance although they can be quite dangerous. In addition, few people are deficient in growth hormone or testosterone, so when athletes take sex steroids or growth hormone hat cheating, or doping.

Vitamin D will improve athletic performance in vitamin D deficient people (and that includes most people). If you are vitamin D deficient, medical literature indicates that the right amount of vitamin D with make you faster, stronger, improve your balance and timing. How much it will improve your athletic ability depends on how deficient you are to begin with. How good an athlete you will be depends on your innate ability, training and dedication.

Sunlight Makes Exercise More Effective

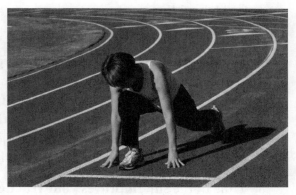

Ancient Greek athletes believed that sunlight "feeds the muscles." They would exercise nude to get the most from their exertions. Now modern science has backed them up. In fact, many studies show that when you exercise in the sun, you get more benefit from exactly the same exercise.

1. **Resting heart rate decreases** and returns to normal following exercise much more rapidly for people who include sunbathing in their fitness regimen.[1]

2. **Respiratory rate decreases after sun exposure.** Breathing is slower, deeper, and easier.[2]

3. **Less lactic acid accumulates** in athletes who get sun exposure. This helps prevent cramping and muscle pain.

4. Several studies have shown that **vitamin D greatly improves lung function.** In fact, one study published in the journal, *Chest*, showed that smokers with the highest levels of vitamin D had better lung function than non-smokers with the lowest levels of vitamin D.

5. Sunlight **increases the ability of blood to carry oxygen** to the tissues. The rise in the oxygen content of the blood following just one exposure to UV light lasts for several days, increasing energy and endurance.[3]

6. A study done on sunlight's effect on carbohydrate metabolism showed an **increase in glycogen stores in the muscles** and liver following sun exposure. Increasing glycogen stores raises energy and endurance.[4]

7. Sun exposure **helps you achieve peak physical condition**. Two studies analyzing the physical fitness of athletes found that peak physical condition happens most commonly in summer months. Your physical condition declines during the winter.[5] One study found that subjects could do more pushups during the summer months than in the winter.[6]

8. Time in the sun **improves your reaction time.** [7] Research also proves that vitamin D supplementation provides significant benefit to functional performance, reaction time and balance.[8]

Dr. Herbert Shelton notes that in times past, all athletes used sunbathing as a regular part of training. In his health-improvement book written more than 70 years ago, he wrote that, *"Muscles subjected to proper sun exposure grow larger, firmer, and have their contractile powers enhanced even without exercise..."*

Accelerate Your Fat Loss with Sunshine

Sunlight helps decrease subcutaneous fat, and improves muscle definition. Sunlight also stimulates the thyroid gland, which increases your metabolism helping you to burn more fat.

People with a vitamin D deficiency are more likely to be obese and obese people are more likely to be vitamin D deficient.[9] This can trap people in a vicious cycle. The more obese they become the worse their deficiency gets which, in turn, makes them even more obese.[10]

Say Hello to Sunshine and Good-bye to Fat

In addition to increasing the effectiveness of exercise, sunshine works in several other ways to help you lose weight.

- **Increase your muscles** – Sunlight improves muscle building. Muscle is your body's biggest metabolic engine. Bigger muscles raise your metabolic rate, and burn more calories even while you're resting.
- **Stimulates production of MSH** – Melanocyte Stimulating Hormone (MSH) has been shown to stimulate weight loss and energy production.
- **Reduces your appetite** – Sunshine causes the body to produce serotonin. Too little serotonin can cause mood swings, carbohydrate cravings and even depression – all associated with weight gain.

Sunlight Makes Your Muscles Stronger

There's more to good fitness than physical activity and a healthy body weight. Muscle strength also plays a role. Both your muscles and bones need vitamin D.

Sunlight increases the oxygen content of blood. It also increases blood supply to the muscles.[11] Likewise, a vitamin D deficiency can cause or worsen conditions that result in the loss of muscle tissue. Examples include myopathy and sarcopenia.[12] [13]

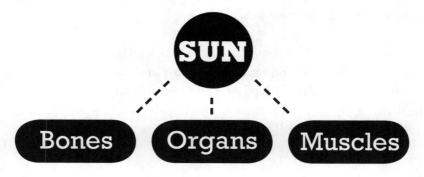

Sunlight Builds Stronger Bones and Teeth

The United States leads the world in dairy consumption, yet our rate of hip fractures and osteoporosis is among the highest in the world. Doctors and researchers are beginning to realize that our nationwide fear of the sun is a big part of the problem.

Bone diseases and fractures are signs of a vitamin D deficiency. Your bones need more than just calcium. Without vitamin D, your body can't use calcium to strengthen its bones. Remember, vitamin D aids in the absorption of calcium from the intestines. Without vitamin D, calcium from your diet never reaches your bones.

From a Wheelchair to Totally Mobile in Six Weeks

In an article titled, *The Miracle of Vitamin D,* nutritionist Krispin Sullivan reports the results of a medical study where "…five patients confined to wheelchairs with severe weakness and fatigue. Blood tests revealed that all suffered from severe vitamin D deficiency. The patients received 50,000 IU vitamin D per week and all became mobile within six weeks."[14]

Vitamin D Deficiency Saps Bone Health

When you have a vitamin D deficiency, 85 percent of the calcium in your food passes straight through your intestines without being absorbed into your body.[15]

Vitamin D regulates other minerals as well like phosphorus and magnesium that your bones need to grow and stay strong. Without vitamin D, you will develop bone loss even if you have enough of these minerals. You must have both vitamin D *and* a proper mineral balance for optimal bone health.

Why Don't Bones get Better with Age?

Studies show that sunshine and vitamin D supplementation by older adults reduces the risk of a broken hip by more than 70 percent. But the older you get the more vitamin D you need, and few get enough.

Let's look more closely at the dangers of vitamin D deficiency as it relates to bone health:

1. **Vitamin D deficiency breaks bones** – In one Minnesota study, researchers examined the vitamin D levels of 78 elderly patients who suffered fragility fractures. Their bones didn't break from trauma; they became so weak they broke with normal daily activities.[16] All 78 of these elders were vitamin D deficient! 80 percent were severely deficient, even though half of them took vitamin D supplements! The researchers concluded that they were not getting enough sunlight or vitamin D to maintain healthy blood levels.

2. **Vitamin D deficiency increases risks of serious falls** – Vitamin D deficiency impairs neuromuscular function, increasing your risk of falling. This puts already weak bones at higher risk for fractures. In many cases, these falls lead to debilitation and death. Fractures lead to a loss of independent living status for more than half of victims. [17]

3. **Vitamin D supplement reduces falls by 30-40 percent** – Research at Creighton University Medical Center in Omaha reveals that vitamin D improves muscle strength and balance in elders. [18] This means fewer falls in addition to stronger bones. Another recent study shows that higher levels of vitamin D are correlated with better walking speed, more balance and greater muscle strength in the elderly.[19]

Common Bone Disorders and Sunlight		
Disease	**Effects**	**Link with Vitamin D**
Rickets	Children's disease: bones soften and bow.	Direct result of severe vitamin D deficiency.
Osteomalacia	Adult's disease: bones become soft and painful.	Severe vitamin D deficiency causes calcium to be pulled from the bones.
Osteoporosis	Adult disease: bones become brittle and fragile. They lose mass.	Adequate vitamin D helps prevent the condition.
Fractures	Broken bones resulting from falls or fragility.	Vitamin D builds both bone strength and balance reducing falls.

Keep a Healthful, Beautiful Smile without Cavities

Teeth are similar to bones. They have nerves and blood feeds them nutrients. And just like your bones, the evidence shows that sun exposure promotes tooth health in several ways:

- **UV-B radiation produced five times fewer cavities** – Researchers fed two groups of hamsters a diet to produce cavities. They raised one group under fluorescent lights and raised the other group under full spectrum lights. The hamsters under the fluorescent lights developed five times as many cavities.[20]

- **Clear correlation between sunlight and tooth decay** – A large study of 94,000 white males between 12 and 14 years found that those who lived in the Northeast, had 65 percent more cavities than those who lived in the Southwest.[21]

- **Cavities higher during the winter and spring** – Another study of 800 children found that cavities were higher during the winter and spring than summer. A study of 90,000 boys showed that cavities were directly related to the amount of sunlight received. Those with the least exposure had double the rate of cavities.[22]

> ## Want to Skip the Dentist's Drill?
>
> Teeth require nutrients for growth and repair. In the wrong environment they break down, becoming weak and vulnerable to infection. Vitamin D helps keep teeth cavity free.

- **Vitamin D deficiency linked to gum disease** – Inflammation can be a leading cause of gum disease and tooth loss. According to the Boston University Dental School, a study of more than 11,000 men and women showed that low blood concentrations of vitamin D were linked to gum disease and tooth loss.

Your Eyes Need to Soak in the Sun

We're told that the sun is a hazard to our eyes. But is it? You might think your eyes' sole function is to turn visible light into images. But your eyes actually are responsible for so much more.

All the blood in your body circulates through the eyes every two hours. As the blood passes through the eyes, they are nourished, but that's not all that happens. Nutrients within the blood itself are actually activated by light.

Should You Wear sunglasses?

Many sunglasses have been developed to specifically block up to 99 percent of UV rays. But these are the essential rays that help us sleep and feel good and are help us to maintain good health.

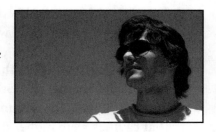

Dr. John Ott, a photobiologist and pioneer in the research of light and health, showed that different parts of the visible spectrum significantly affected different biological responses. He also found that cells in the eyes of rabbits would only divide if exposed to low levels of UV light.

Dr. Jacob Liberman, optometrist and author of the book *Light: Medicine of the Future*, also writes that our indoor lifestyle combined with "excessive use of sunglasses" inhibit normal cell division by blocking UV light and increase the number of cases of macular degeneration.[25]

Cataract Controversy

Many eye doctors blame the sun for cataracts because sunny locations have greater rates. But there has been a dramatic increase in modern times yet the sun doesn't shine more now than it did in the past.

In fact, exposure to sunlight through your eyes may help to prevent cataracts and macular degeneration. The risk of cataracts in elders goes down with optimal vitamin D.[23] There is also strong evidence linking increases in cataracts to other causes like poor nutrition, smoking, and pollution. We do know that those who consume a nutritious diet rarely get cataracts, regardless of how much sun exposure they have.[24]

Solar Powered Fitness

The Pineal Gland: Your Internal Light Meter

The pineal gland is a tiny pea-shaped gland that is positioned behind the eyes and is sometimes called the "third eye." The pineal gland serves as your light meter, communicating to the body what season it is and whether it is night or day. It keeps you connected to the rhythms of nature.

The main functions of the pineal gland are to produce melatonin and serotonin. These are two neurotransmitters that directly influence brain function and your entire endocrine system. But the pineal gland needs the cycles of sunlight and darkness to do this properly. In turn, it also cycles hormone production by the hypothalamus gland as well.[26]

The hypothalamus controls many of your life sustaining functions including your nervous system, fluid balance, heat regulation, circulation and breathing. The pineal and hypothalamus glands both directly influence sexual function.[27] In this sense, the pineal gland is like the master conductor and the hypothalamus is the high command center. And both are directly affected by the light that enters your eyes.[28]

Without sufficient melatonin produced by the pineal gland, we are more susceptible to cancer. Without enough stimulus from sunlight, the pineal gland can become calcified and produce less melatonin.

There are many stories that correlate the excessive use of sunglasses with cancer. There have also been anecdotal cases of "spontaneous remission" soon after patients discarded their glasses and began to enjoy the rays of the healing sun.[29]

Weight Gain in the Winter – Pineal and Hunger

Then of course, who has never complained of weight gain in winter and taken refuge behind the excuse that your body needs extra fat reserves during the cold months? Well, that may be partly true, but if your pineal gland is not exposed to sufficient natural light during the day, you are likely to have a ravenous appetite and, with your appetite out of control, you simply cannot hope to manage your weight effectively.

Sunlight Balances Your Hormones

The sun regulates a number of hormones in your body, including those that work as part of the stress response, and those that control your endocrine system, biological clock, and immune system. The 24-hour cycle of light and dark is vital in the production and regulation of hormones.

It's not your willpower or your occupation that controls your circadian rhythm – it is your hormones. The sun regulates these hormones, stimulating them with light.[30]

Sunlight	Result in your body
Triggers a release of melatonin	Reduces UV-induced free radicals
Stimulates your hypothalamus to produce serotonin	Helps you stay positive and mentally healthy
Suppresses the pineal gland's production of melatonin at night	Sets your biological clock
Causes the pituitary to stimulate the endocrine system	Regulates numerous other hormones in the body

Melatonin can function as an anti-oxidant and free radical scavenger. Sunlight triggers a release of melatonin, reducing UV-induced free radicals. This is another self-regulating part of nature; exposure to the sun can cause free radicals, but it also produces a response in your body to deal with them.[31]

Relieve Premenstrual Syndrome (PMS) with Sunlight

Sunlight and vitamin D are also involved in PMS and it is known that lower vitamin D and calcium levels increases symptoms of PMS:

- A large study of female nurses beginning in 1989 followed women over time to determine the links between diet, life-style and disease. Researchers found that the women with the most vitamin D and calcium in their diet were half as likely to experience the symptoms of PMS.[32]

- Another study showed that vitamin D, calcium and magnesium together were able to eliminate the symptoms of PMS.[33] This Study also suggested that PMS is really a "calcium deficiency state that is unmasked" by the rise in hormones during the menstrual cycle.

The Healing Action of Sunshine

Research has found that exposure to sunlight may influence the healing process for a large variety of ailments:

- **Open wounds and broken bones** – Dr. Carl Hoffminster wrote that soldiers healed and survived better when their wounds and broken bones were exposed to sunlight. He also noticed it kept wounds germ free and healed infections.

- **Wounds heal faster** – When NASA studied the use of infrared light therapy, they found that it helped wounds heal up to 200 percent faster.

- **Back pain is improved** – Vitamin D deficiency is a major contributor to chronic low back pain. In one study that when vitamin D was administered to patients with unexplained back pain, 95 percent experienced an improvement in their symptoms.

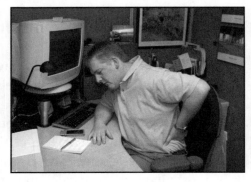

- **Less pain medication** – Researchers in Pennsylvania studied the effects of sunlight on spinal surgery outcomes. Patients on the bright side of the hospital usede 22 percent less pain medication than patients on the shady side of the hospital.[34]

- **Chronic pain, muscular weakness and fatigue** – Swiss researchers found that patients with chronic pain, muscular weakness and fatigue were almost always vitamin D deficient. When treated with supplemental vitamin D, the patients saw a complete resolution of their condition, usually within three months.[35]

Check out this chart for a peek into some of sunlight's numerous other health benefits:

Detoxification	Sunlight helps your body to detoxify, speeding up the elimination of harmful chemicals. Studies have shown that sunlight helps animals expel lead, mercury, cobalt, manganese, cadmium, fluoride, pesticides, and dusts from their system 10 to 20 times faster than those without light.
Digestive Health	Research has shown links between low blood levels of vitamin D, ulcerative colitis and Chrohn's disease.
Gout	Gout occurs due to a uric acid buildup in the body. Sun helps the body excrete uric acid, in turn decreasing the occurrence of gout.
Hearing	Vitamin D deficiency can also cause hearing loss in elders. This is caused by the cochlea bone in the inner ear becoming more porous.
Stress	Sunlight calms mood and relieves stomach ulcers. A number of studies show that sunlight improves ulcer symptoms and can prevent them from re-occurring.[36]
Sleep	Sunlight is essential for healthy sleeping and waking cycles. It regulates your circadian rhythm and can cure sleeping problems. It stimulates the suppression and production of melatonin, your sleep hormone.

Plan to Enjoy the Sun Year Round

As you can see from this chapter, it is absolutely vital to your health and your enjoyment of life that you get enough sunlight and vitamin D.

In the summer, plan to do something outside every day. Here are some ideas:

- Go hiking
- Visit a farmer's market
- Picnic in the park
- Play Frisbee with friends
- Visit a local lake or river for a swim
- Play a game of basketball with a buddy
- Kick a soccer ball around with your grandkids
- If all else fails… just take a walk!

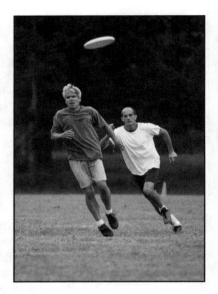

Remember, in the summer less clothing is better if you're not going to be in the sun for a long time all at once. You'll maximize your vitamin D production by exposing your skin.

In the winter, you should boost the benefit of your indoor exercise with vitamin D if you live in a northern climate. And, you should still try and get outside and exercise in the sunlight whenever you can.

On work days, make a commitment to taking a walk at lunch on any day that the sun is out. On winter weekends, get outside for walks, visits to the park, or play in the snow when the sun is out.

(Endnotes)

1 Kime, ZR. (1980). *Sunlight*. Penryn, CA: World Health Publications. p. 34.

Solar Powered Fitness

2 Laurens, H. (1939). The Physiologic Effect of Ultraviolet Radiation. *JAMA*. 11:2385.

3 Miley, G. (1939). Ultraviolet Blood Radiation: Studies in Oxygen Absorption. *American Journal of Medical Science.* 197:873.

4 Pincussen, L. (1937). The Effect of Ultraviolet and Visible Rays on Carbohydrate Metabolism, Arch Phys Ther X-Ray Radium. 18:750.

5 Kwarecki, K. (1981). Circannual rhythms of physical fitness and tolerance of hypoxic hypoxia. *Acta Physiol Pol.* 32(6):629-36.

6 Koch, H, et al. (2000). Circannual period of physical performance analysed by means of standard cosinor analysis: a case report. *Rom J Physiol.* 37(1-4-):51-8.

7 Dhesi, JK, et al. (2004). Vitamin D supplementation improves neuromuscular function in older people who fall. Age Ageing. 33(6):589-95.

8 Dhesi, JK, et al. (2002). Neuromuscular and psychomotor function in elderly subjects who fall and the relationship with vitamin D status. *J Bone Miner Res.* 17(5):891-7.

9 Shi, H, et al. (2001). 1alpha,25-Dihydroxyvitamin D3 modulates human adipocyte metabolism via nongenomic action. *FASEB J.* 15(14):2751-3.

10 Wortsman, J, et al. (2000). Decreased bioavailability of vitamin D in obesity. *Am J Clin Nutr.* 72(3):690-3.

11 Kime, ZR. (1980). *Sunlight*. Penryn, CA: World Health Publications. p. 36.

12 Prabhala, A, et al. (2000). Severe myopathy associated with vitamin D deficiency in western New York. *Arch.Intern.Med.* 160:1199-203.

13 Visser, M, et al. (2003). Low vitamin D and high parathyroid hormone levels as determinants of loss of muscle strength and muscle mass (sarcopenia): the Longitudinal Aging Study Amsterdam. *J Clin Endocrinol Metab.* 88(12):5766-72.

14 Sullivan, K. The Miracle of Vitamin D. The Weston A. Price Foundation. http://www.westonaprice.org/basicnutrition/vitamindmiracle.html

15 Holick, MF. (2004). Vitamin D: importance in the prevention of cancers, type 1 diabetes, heart disease, and osteoporosis. *Am J Clin Nutr.* 79(3):362-71.

16 Simonelli, C, et al. (2005). Prevalence of vitamin D inadequacy in a minimal trauma fracture population. *Curr Med Res Opin.* 21(7):1069-74.

17 Kenzora JE, et al. " Hip Fracture Mortality: Relation to Age, Treatment, Pre-operative Illness, Time of Surgery, and Complications," *Clinical Orthopaedics* 1984; 186: 45-56

18 Gallagher, JC. (2004). The effects of calcitriol on falls and fractures and physical performance tests. *J Steroid Biochem Mol Biol.* 89-90(1-5):497-501.

19 Bischoff-Ferrari, HA. (2004). Effect of Vitamin D on falls: a meta-analysis. *JAMA.* 291(16):1999-2006.

20 Sharon, IM, et al. (1971). The Effects of Lights of Different Spectra on Caries Incidence in the Golden Hamster. *Archives of Oral Biology.* 16(12):1427-1431.

21 Hobday, R. (1999). *The Healing Sun: Sunlight and Health in the 21st Century.* Scotland: Findhorn Press. p. 80.

22 East, BR. (1939). Mean Annual Hours of Sunshine and the Incidence of Dental Caries. *Amer J Public Health.* 29:777.

23 Jacques, PF, et al. (1988). Nutritional status in persons with and without senile cataract: blood vitamin and mineral levels. *Am J Clin Nutr.* 48:152-8.

24 Best, S. Here comes the sun – get out in it! Caduceus. http://www.caduceus.info/articles/best.htm

25 Liberman, J. (1991). *Light: Medicine of the Future.* Sante Fe, NM: Bear & Company. p. 150.

26 Faigin, R. *Natural Hormonal Enhancement.* Cedar Mountain, NC: Extique Publishing. P. 203.

27 Wallen, EP, et al. (1987). Photoperiodic response in the male laboratory rat. *Biol Reprod.* 37:22.

28 Liberman, J. (1991). *Light: Medicine of the Future.* Rochester, VT: Bear & Company. p. 25.

29 Osborne, SE. Seeing the Light. Price-Pottenger Nutrition Foundation. http://www.price-pottenger.org/Articles/SeeingTheLight.html

30 Duffy, JF, et al. (1996). Phase-shifting human circadian rhythms: influence of sleep timing, social contact, and light exposure. *J Physiol (Lond).* 495:289.

31 Fischer, TW, et al. (2001). Melatonin reduces UV-induced reactive oxygen species in a dose-dependent manner in IL-3-stimulated leukocytes. *J Pineal Res.* 31(1):39-45.

32 Bertone-Johnson, ER, et al. (2005). Calcium and vitamin D intake and risk of incident premenstrual syndrome. *Arch Intern Med.* 165:1246-1252.

33 Thys-Jacobs, S. (2000). Micronutrients and the premenstrual syndrome: the case for calcium. *J Am Coll Nutr.* 19:220-7.

34 Elias, M. (2004). Sunlight reduces need for pain medication. USA Today, March 2, 2004. http://www.usatoday.com/news/health/2004-03-02-sunlight-pain_x.htm

35 de la Jara, GT, Pécoud, A, Favrat, B. Musculoskeletal pain in female asylum seekers and hypovitaminosis D3. BMJ. 2004 Jul 17;329(7458):156-7

36 Kime, ZR. (1980). *Sunlight.* Penryn, CA: World Health Publications. p. 4.

CHAPTER TWELVE

Brighten Up Your Winter

*"Do not anticipate trouble or worry about what
may never happen. Keep in the sunlight."*

– Benjamin Franklin

E very winter, about 25 percent of the population suffers a significant decline in their mood and energy. We often call it the
winter blues.

Of those suffering with winter blues, more than 20 percent develop full-blown depression tied to the season.[1] This phenomenon
is called seasonal affective disorder, or SAD. Reduced visible light
striking the eye and sunlight striking the skin cause SAD.

The light that strikes the eyes is extremely important, but so is
the vitamin D that is created when sunlight strikes your skin. This
is backed up by the fact that vitamin D supplementation can successfully treat SAD. The fact that seasonal affective disorder is more
common as you move away from the equator – the same pattern
that vitamin D decline follows in winter months – is yet more evidence that vitamin D plays a role.

Get a little sadder in the winter? You're not alone!

- Seasonal changes can cause clinical winter depression in approx
  6 percent of the population.
- Up to 25 percent of the population gets the "winter blues."
  Symptoms include increased intake of carbohydrates, longer
  sleep patterns, lethargy, fatigue, irritability, lowered motivation
  and decreased sociability. Remission comes in spring.

There is plenty of evidence to show that SAD is connected with the amount of sunlight you get during winter months. For example:

1. **SAD causes carbohydrate cravings** – Carb cravings are a well-documented symptom of SAD and depression.[2] Low serotonin levels can cause cravings for carbohydrates. Sunlight causes your body to produce serotonin that elevates your mood and reduces your craving for carbs.

2. **SAD is most common where winters are long and dark** – SAD is most common in Norway and Finland. The winters that far north are long and dark – sometimes there is only three hours worth of daylight. SAD increases fatigue, illness, insomnia, depression, alcoholism, and suicide.

3. **Vitamin D relieves SAD symptoms** – In clinical trials, vitamin D relieved depression more effectively than broad-spectrum light exposure.[3]

You Can Beat SAD and Enjoy Your Winter

The best way to conquer SAD would be finding a way to spend time in natural sunlight. But even if this isn't possible there are several other ways you can increase your vitamin D stores and decrease your struggles with SAD.

Phototherapy is effective at treating SAD and can even be used to treat non-seasonal depression. Phototherapy involves regular exposure to bright lights through a light box. Phototherapy uses very bright lights that approximate the spectrum of daylight much better than most indoor lighting.

People with SAD can use a light box for 30 minutes to two hours a day during the winter. If they are bright enough and produce the UVB part of the light spectrum, these lights can even help produce vitamin D.

Dawn Simulation – In another study researchers found that using a morning alarm that simulates a late spring dawn was helpful to those who suffer from SAD. These alarms use full-spectrum light that slowly brightens a room to simulate the rising sun. In this study, the device helped relieve SAD symptoms in 49 percent of cases.[4]

Negative Air Ionization – The same researchers who looked at dawn simulation also tested using high-flow air ionization that negatively charged air molecules in the hour and half before waking. This treatment was effective 48 percent of the time.

Vitamin D supplementation – Phototherapy is an effective treatment for many people, but it doesn't work for everyone. An even better solution is to also supplement with vitamin D. In one study that compared vitamin D supplementation with two-hour daily use of light boxes, the symptoms of depression in the vitamin D group were resolved completely, while the light therapy group saw no significant improvement in symptoms.[5]

Treat Depression with Sunshine

Everyone has sad days, or even weeks, here and there. If you have never experienced real depression, it can be difficult to understand why someone cannot just "snap out of it." Clinical depression is much more than just a feeling – it has a biochemical basis. And the number of people diagnosed with depression is on the rise.

Several large studies show that there have been sweeping changes in the rates of major depression in developed countries in the last century. This increase coincides with populations moving from the country into the city, working in buildings, traveling in cars and using more sunscreen.[6] As people get less sun, the rates of depression are surging.

Less Sun, More Depression

There is a clear association between reduced sun exposure and increased incidence of depression. And vitamin D deficiency is a significant factor in clinical depression. There is a clear association between low vitamin D levels and the symptoms of depression.

Could Depression be a Sign That I'm Deficient in Vitamin D?

Studies show that as vitamin D levels decline, symptoms of depression increase. On the other hand, as vitamin D levels increase, symptoms of depression decrease. The answer is yes! Vitamin D supplementation is a great place to start fighting off depression.

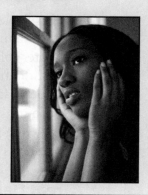

Our world revolves around the sun and, quite literally, the sun will make you shine!

Fight Back Against Depression with More Light and More Vitamin D

There are two components to SAD – your body misses the bright full-spectrum light entering your eyes and stimulating the pineal gland <u>and</u> it misses the vitamin D synthesis that sunlight triggers in your skin.

You can fight back in a number of ways.

First, go outside more during the winter. Whenever the sun is out, make a point to spend some time outside. The full-spectrum, natural light of the sun is unparalleled when it comes to light therapy. It's especially good to go out and play in the snow – there is a lower incidence of SAD in regions that get regular amounts of snow, probably because the snow reflects light and brightens up the world.

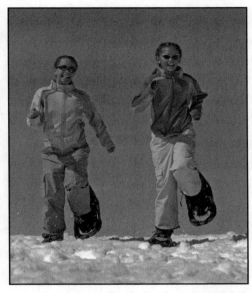

Second, look into a natural light alarm to wake you in the morning. These alarms can make a big difference in how refreshed you feel throughout the day… and they can fight SAD, too.

Third, make sure you take a vitamin D supplement during the winter months.

Finally, pay attention to your moods and limitations. SAD unfortunately strikes during the holiday season, and that can compound how you are feeling. Don't feel obligated to accept every invitation to every party you receive or undertake every task you are asked to do. Instead, learn to say "no" politely, but firmly.

Don't overdo it on the sugary foods and alcoholic beverages that are prevalent during the early winter months – they can make you feel worse. Seek help if you need it – there's no shame in talking to a counselor, and it can be very productive.

By being proactive, you can fight back against seasonal depression and begin to enjoy winter… and the holidays… just like you did when you were young.

(Endnotes)

1 "Seasonal Affective Disorder." Information provided by St. Louis Psychologists and Counseling Information and Referral Services.

2 Ghadirian, AM, et al. (1999). Seasonal mood patterns in eating disorders. Gen Hosp Psychiatry. 21:354.

3 Gloth, FM, et al. (1999). Vitamin D vs broad spectrum phototherapy in the treatment of seasonal affective disorder. J Nutr Health Aging. 3:5-7.

4 Terman M and Terman JS (2006) Controlled trial of naturalistic dawn simulation and negative air ionization for seasonal affective disorder, Am J Psychiatry, 163(12): 2126-33

5 Gloth, FM, et al. (1999). Vitamin D vs broad spectrum phototherapy in the treatment of seasonal affective disorder. J Nutr Health Aging. 3:5-7.

6 Klerman, GL, Weissman, MM. (1989). Increasing rates of depression. JAMA. 261(15):2229-35.

CHAPTER THIRTEEN

Light-up Your Sex Life

*"The sun, the hearth of affection and life, pours
burning love on the delighted earth."*

– Arthur Rimbaud

Free from side effects and costs, sunlight can effectively boost
your sex drive and fertility and even improve your sexual performance. Sunlight can also lessen the impact of aging on your
sexual health.

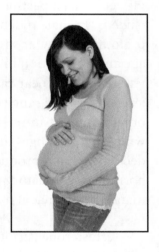

As you will soon see, sunlight is important to other aspects of sexual health as
well, like sexual hormone production and
reproductive health. New research finds that
a pregnant mother's vitamin D level impacts
the long-term health of her future children
influencing everything from their height and
weight to their academic ability.[1]

And, you'll be delighted to enjoy the
many healthy and pleasurable benefits from
reigniting your oldest, safest and most effective aphrodisiac.

Natural Hormone Enhancement

It turns out that there is more going on at the beach to sexually
excite us than skimpy bathing suites. Sun exposure directly aids
and boosts testosterone production - the main hormone of sexual
desire in both men and women.

Men have about 15 times more testosterone than women do. This extra testosterone in men helps to shape the male physique, keep men strong, and is largely responsible for a man's sex drive and potency. It also increases a man's energy and mental acuity.

Interestingly, it makes a difference where the sunlight hits your body. For instance, there is a bigger boost in testosterone production when sunlight strikes the male genitals. One study, performed in the 1930s showed that, "When the chest or back is exposed to sunlight, the male hormones may increase by 120%. When the genital area is exposed, the hormones can increase by 200%."[2]

In *Natural Hormonal Enhancement*, author Rob Faigin reviewed sixteen pertinent peer reviewed animal studies and concluded: "In male rodents, experimental light deprivation causes profound testicular shrinkage and a reduction in testosterone levels to near castrate levels. In a wide range of other animals, summer to winter light changes induce decrements in reproductive hormones, copulatory performance, and gonadal mass"

Testosterone isn't just for men... women need it, too. The good news is that the sun also boosts sex hormones in women. In addition to testosterone, estrogen absorption also increases when a woman gets some sun exposure.[3]

Can Sunlight Decrease the Effects of Aging on my Sex Drive?

For both men and women, age can cause deficiencies of sex hormones, leading to a decrease in sexual performance and libido. Sunlight is an effective way to help your body overcome this and rebuild more youthful hormone levels.

Get to bed early and rise early in the morning to maximize your daylight hours. Then get out the door. The boost is fast – you may feel improved sexual performance that very night.

Light-up Your Sex Life

More Babies Are Made in Summer

Regular exposure to sunlight helps to balances the reproductive hormones (oestrogen, testosterone and progesterone) and has a positive effect on fertility, impotence and can improve ovulation irregularities.

There is a seasonal distribution in conception and birth rates. In northern countries, the conception rate decreases during the winter and peaks during the summer. It's likely that seasonal influences on female ovulation play an important role.[4]

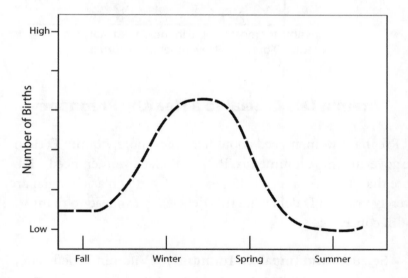

Lower rates of conception in winter could also result from lower vitamin D levels during the dark winter months:

- In a study on the reproductive effects of Vitamin D, researchers found that male rats with vitamin D deficiency had 45 percent lower ability to reproduce than male rats with optimal vitamin D levels.[5]

- Another study of rats found that deficiency of vitamin D also reduces sperm count.[6]

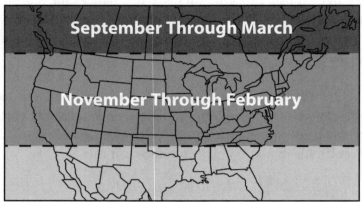

It's not possible for most people in the United States to get vitamin D between November and February.

Vitamin D is Crucial to a Healthy Pregnancy

Pregnant women need about ten times more vitamin D than the government recommends. Pregnant black women need a lot more than that. As a result, 12 percent of young black women are severely vitamin D deficient. This deficiency can lead to many health concerns:

- **Seizures and Impaired Immunity** – Vitamin D deficiency in the mother can be linked to seizures in children and impaired immune function.[7]
- **Severe deficiency can lead to serious brain damage** – In a rat model, Australian researchers found that even transient deficiencies during gestation can cause permanent brain damage.[8] Other studies have confirmed these findings.[9] In the more complex human brain this would cause lifelong consequences on learning, personality, memory and IQ.

Light-up Your Sex Life

These patterns have never been observed in tropical areas, where there is minimal climate difference in the summer and winter. A study of Hawaiian children without seasonal sun variation shows no difference in these factors of learning and behavior between children born at different times of the year.

Vitamin D Status of the Pregnant Mother Has a Long-Term Impact on the Height of the Child

Expecting mothers are more vitamin D deficient during the winter months and in colder climates where they have less exposure to the sun. And recent studies have found that the time of year in which a child is born may have lasting effects on growth and development:

- Studies show that there is a connection between what month of the year a child is born and how tall that child will become.

- A study published in Early Human Development confirms that the amount of sunlight a mother gets during pregnancy is the most significant factor

Does the time of year I was born affect my academic abilities?

The vitamin D status of pregnant mothers seems to have a strong influence on the academic abilities (and behavior patterns) of children. When asked about this, Dr. John Cannell of the Vitamin D Council points to a Harvard study, which showed that summer-born boys were seven times more likely to have learning disabilities.[10] (In summer born children, the early development of the brain occurs in winter.)

A University of Georgia review of the literature confirmed these results, stating that summer born children were "more frequently retained, performed lower on standardized tests, and were more frequently diagnosed with specific learning disabilities."[11]

determining the future height of the child. Researchers measured these children at birth and then followed them to the age of two.[12]

Natural Sexual and Reproductive Health

If the sun can lift our mood, lessen our depression and increase our immunity, it seems obvious that it would also have great effect on our sexuality and reproduction. We are just now beginning to understand the ramifications of being vitamin D deficient, especially during pregnancy. Perhaps more than any other area, pregnancy also highlights the vast impact that raising our overall vitamin D levels could make on our health and well-being as a society.

Get Naked in the Sun!

Before you learn about the best way to

More than half of women suffer vitamin D deficiency during pregnancy

More than half of pregnant women today do not have sufficient amounts of vitamin D, even with prenatal vitamin supplements as part of their regimen, a new University of Pittsburgh study shows. The study found that more than 80 percent of African-American women and nearly half of the Caucasian women tested at delivery had levels of vitamin D that were way too low.

More than 90 percent of the women in the study used prenatal vitamins, but still did not have enough vitamin D.

Vitamin D helps fights rickets, a disease that softens the bones. Rickets is among the most frequent childhood diseases in many developing countries and has been making a comeback in America among infants.

The daily recommended intake of vitamin D – 400 IUs – is insufficient for disease prevention, especially during pregnancy.

Light-up Your Sex Life

light your house in the next chapter, give this fun activity a try. You'll have to step outside your comfort zone, but you'll find the benefits are worth it.

Remember, earlier in this chapter you learned that sun striking the male genitals can trigger a significantly greater response in sex hormone production. Well, this summer, find somewhere appropriate and at least twice a month enjoy the sunlight naked.

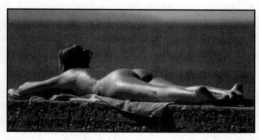

This task is easier if you have a private, fenced backyard. But even if you don't, you can still give this a try. You can either visit a local beach that allows nude sunbathing. Or you can go backpacking where few people go. Chances are you'll find a secluded river or lake where you'll feel comfortable in your birthday suit.

Try to get naked in the sunshine... at least occasionally!

One word of caution, your skin surrounding the genitals may be extra sensitive to sunlight since it gets so little exposure. Don't overdo it. It's the last place you want a sunburn.

Read on to the next chapter to find out what kind of natural lighting causes less hyperactivity for children and better concentration for all of us.

(Endnotes)

1 Morley R, et al. "Maternal 25-hydroxyvitamin D and parathyroid hormone concentrations and offspring birth size," *J Clin Endocrinol Metab* 2006; 91(3): 906-12

2 Myerson, A, and Neustadt, R. (1930). Influence of ultraviolet irradiation upon excretion of sex hormones in the male. *Endocrinolgy*. 25:7.

3 Lieberman, J. (1991). *Light: Medicine of the Future*. Rochester, VT: Bear & Company.

4 Rojansky, N, et al. (1992). Seasonality in human reproduction: an update. *Hum Reprod*. (6):735-45.

5 Kwiecinski, GG, et al. (1989). Vitamin D is necessary for reproductive functions of the male rat. *J Nutr*. 119(5):741-4.

6 Sood, S, et al. (1992). Effect of vitamin D deficiency on testicular function in the rat. *Ann Nutr Metab*. 36(4):203-8.

7 Dijkstra SH, et al. "Seizures in foreign newborns due to maternal vitamin-D deficiency," *Ned Tijdschr Geneeskd* 2005; 149(5): 257-60

8 Feron F, et al. (2005). Developmental vitamin D3 deficiency alters the adult rat brain. *Brain Res Bull*. 65(2):141-8.

9 Eyles, D, et al. (2003). Vitamin D and brain development. *Neuroscience*. 118(3):641-53.

10 Badian, NA. (1984). Reading disability in an epidemiological context incidence and environmental correlates.
J Learn Disabil. 17(3):129-36.

11 Martin, RP, et al. (2004). Season of birth is related to child retention rates, achievement, and rate of diagnosis of specific LD. *J Learn Disabil*. 37(4):307-17.

12 Mercola.com. Let the sun shine in (especially when pregnant). http://www.mercola.com

CHAPTER FOURTEEN

Choose the Right Indoor Lights for Health

"The light of the body is your eye; when your eye is clear, your whole body is clear, your whole body is also full of light; but when it is bad, your body is full of darkness."

– Luke 11:34, The Bible

Many of us spend all our waking hours under lights that don't mimic sunlight. There's a drawback to being inside under artificial light all day. Most indoor lights do not give us the UV energy we are meant to flourish under.

Fortunately, there's something that you can do right now in your office space or home to improve your health and immunity. Light bulbs that emit a spectrum similar to that of natural sunlight are available.

And, there are other things you can do to bring sunlight into your indoor spaces. You'll cut down on germs and sickness. You'll improve your vitamin D levels. And, you'll brighten everyone's mood.

What is Full Spectrum Lighting and Why is It Important?

Photobiologists first coined the term full-spectrum in the 1960's to describe electric lights closest to the natural spectrum. These lights simulate the ultraviolet (UV) spectrum of natural sunlight.

Full spectrum light provides a number of health benefits from helping to prevent skin cancer to increasing learning ability and reducing stress.

Fluorescent Lights May Increase Risk of Skin Cancer

Studies implicate fluorescent lighting in the formation of melanoma. This could explain why more office workers get melanoma than do outdoor workers.[1][2] UVC radiation, which the atmosphere normally filters out, is present in some artificial lights. Fluorescent lights may contribute to skin cancer by emitting UVC without atmospheric filtration.

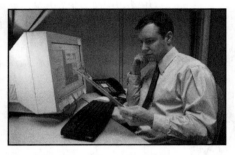

In 1980, German doctor Fritz Hollwich compared the effects of fluorescent and full-spectrum lights on the hormonal system. The fluorescent lights produced high levels of stress hormones in the subjects, while the subjects under full-spectrum lights had normal levels of stress hormones.[3] In Germany, cool-white fluorescent bulbs are actually banned in hospitals and medical facilities based on this research.

Farmed Chickens Get it. How About You?

Chicken farmers now raise their indoor birds under full-spectrum lighting. As a result, the chickens live twice as long, lay more eggs, they are less aggressive to other birds, and their eggs even have 25 percent less cholesterol.

The cholesterol lowering effect of full spectrum lighting is exactly the same for us, yet most of us have yet to change our working conditions. Does it make sense for chickens to reap the benefits of full spectrum lighting while we work under lights linked to cancer?

Choose the Right Indoor Lights for Health

Full-Spectrum Lighting –
A Full Spectrum of Health Benefits

Here is a small sampling of the evidence for the health benefits of full-spectrum lights.

1. **Reduced risk of breast and colon cancer** – A long-term population study conducted by Johns Hopkins University Medical School showed exposure to full-spectrum artificial lighting reduces risk of breast and colon cancer.[4]

2. **Reduced risk of tumors** – Dr. John Ott conducted an experiment in 1964 where mice bred to produce tumors were kept under three different types of light – cool white, pink fluorescent, and full-spectrum. Those under pink lights developed tumors first (after 42 weeks). Those under cool white lights developed tumors after 47 weeks. Under full-spectrum lights, they developed tumors after 51 weeks.[5]

3. **Increased calcium absorption** – Researchers at the Chelsea, Massachusetts Soldiers' Home conducted a study to see if UV light helped veterans absorb more calcium. Since it was winter, they used full-spectrum lights instead of sunlight. The group without UV light showed a 25 percent decrease in calcium absorption. The group with UV light increased calcium absorption by 15 percent. Those with exposure to UV absorbed 40 percent more calcium from the exact same diet.[6]

4. **Less illness in office buildings and schools** – UV full-spectrum lighting reduces illness in office buildings and schools. This is likely due to the anti-virus anti-bacterial properties of UV light.

5. **Less infection after operations** – In 1935, Dr. Deryl Hart of Duke University became disturbed by the number of infections following surgical procedures. Dr. Hart was able to grow 78 different colonies of bacteria in one Petri dish left in an operating room. To remedy the situation, Dr. Hart suspended ultraviolet lights from the ceiling of the operating room. He found the lights were able to kill all the bacteria within 8 feet in less than 10 minutes. This was at a low intensity.[7]

> ## Are fluorescent lights sucking the life out of you?
>
> If you work under cool-white fluorescent lights, you should replace them with full-spectrum lights. You can find them online by doing a search for "full spectrum lights" or at major home improvement and department stores. You may also want to visit www.sperti.com. This company has developed an indoor light box that is especially effective at promoting vitamin D production. Choosing the right indoor lighting is especially important if you are unable to get frequent sun exposure.

6. **Less colds and sore throats** – In Russia, they've used full spectrum lighting in factories for a long time. They found it helps to prevent colds and sore throats among the workers. The low intensity UV exposure reduces bacterial contamination of the air by 40 percent to 70 percent. Their counterparts with no UV light were absent due to sickness twice as much.[8]

7. **Improved immunity** – A study on laboratory workers in Florida showed that there was not one employee that called in sick during the 1968 Hong Kong flu epidemic (these employees had not been inoculated either). However, the company they worked for had installed full spectrum lighting

Choose the Right Indoor Lights for Health

and ultraviolet-transmitting windowpanes. The researchers also noted that the staff were in much better spirits and were more productive in their new workplace.

What Kind of Lights Are Your Children Exposed To?

There is a strong relationship between the type of indoor lighting and the health and learning capabilities of children. In fact, research shows that replacing fluorescent lights with full-spectrum lighting in schools makes a huge difference:

1. **Better growth** – Researchers in Canada examined the ef-

    fects of different types of lighting on the growth of elementary school children. Children attending a school with lights containing UV rays showed the best growth.[9]

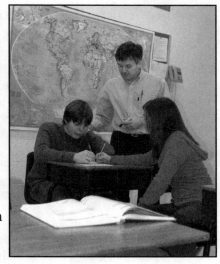

2. **Improved school performance** – In this same study, children attending school under full-spectrum lights also performed better academically.

3. **Less hyperactivity** – The light environment in schools plays a role in children's behavior and learning abilities. Time-lapse photography has been used to show that children became calmer under full-spectrum lights and more hyperactive under normal fluorescent lights.[10]

Bring the Sun into Your Home

When it comes to getting the vitamin D that your body needs, your best source, of course, is natural sunlight. We're just beginning to understand all the benefits of full spectrum lighting and the early research is promising.

If you do have access to sunlight, it makes no sense to continually block yourself from it by "living in sunscreen." In the next chapter, you'll find out why to avoid sunscreen and how to enjoy natural sunlight safely.

Your Children do Better in School with Full Spectrum Lighting

In 1973, Dr. John Ott conducted a study with the Environmental Health and Light Research Institute in first grade classrooms in Sarasota, Florida. In the study, full-spectrum lights were installed in two windowless classrooms. In two identical windowless classrooms, normal fluorescent fixtures were installed.

The researchers then photographed the children intermittently with time-lapse cameras. They found that the children under regular lights showed fatigue and irritability as well as hyperactivity and attention deficit.

On the other hand, the children under full spectrum lights showed better academic performance (their learning and reading improved). They also showed a calmer demeanor and had one third the cavities of the other children.

Assess Your Light at Work and Home

It's easy to take advantage of full-spectrum lighting.

Choose the Right Indoor Lights for Health

Begin by doing a "light audit" of your office space and your home space. What kinds of light bulbs do you use? Are they full spectrum? What about your windows? Are they covered with heavy curtains? Or do you use blinds that make it easy to let light in?

Note how many new full spectrum light bulbs you need to replace your old light bulbs. Write down the kind of bulbs you need (standard lamp, tube bulb, or specialty bulb) and how many of each. Also note the wattage you want. Then go shopping. Your local home improvement store should have what you need. If not, there are many sources for vitamin D lamps and full spectrum light bulbs online.

Next, work on your windows. Are your curtains easy to draw back? Then make a habit of opening them up when you get up in the morning. If not, do some improvements, so that your curtains are either lighter weight or easier to open. Consider adding Venetian blinds to your windows. They make it easy to let in more light.

(Endnotes)

1 Walter, SD, et al. (1992). The association of cutaneous malignant melanoma and fluorescent light exposure.
Am J Epidemio. 135:749.

2 Beral, V, et al. (1982). Malignant melanoma and exposure to fluorescent lighting at work. *Lancet.* 2:290.

3 Hollwich F, Dieckhues B. (1980). The effect of natural and artificial light via the eye on the hormonal and metabolic balance of animal and man. *Opthalmologica.* 180(4):188-197.

4 Goldberg, Burton. *Alternative Medicine.* p305

5 Ott, JN. (1985). Color and light: their effects on plants, animals, and people. *Journal of Biosocial Research 7, part I.*

6 Neer, RM, et al. (1971). <u>Stimulation by artificial lighting of calcium absorption in elderly human subjects.</u> *Nature.* 229:255.

7 Kime, ZR. (1980). *Sunlight.* Penryn, CA: World Health Publications. p. 268.

8 Kime, ZR. (1980). *Sunlight.* Penryn, CA: World Health Publications. p. 169.

9 Hathaway WE, et al. "A Study into the Effects of Light on Children of Elementary School-Age – A Case of Daylight Robbery." Available from Alberta Deprartment of Education. 1992.

10 Ott, J. N. (1976). Influence of fluorescent lights on hyperactivity and learning disabilities. Journal of Learning Disabilities, 2 (7), 417-422.

CHAPTER FIFTEEN

Throw Away Cancer-Causing Sunscreens

"The best protection against skin cancer is a good tan."

– George Hamilton

Using sunscreen on occasion may be better than suffering sunburn. But there is no evidence that they will protect you from skin cancer. In fact, evidence suggests just the opposite – that sunscreens have partially *caused* the increase in skin cancer.

Sunscreens block your skin from producing the pigment melanin. This prevents your body from employing its natural defense against overexposure to sunlight – a tan. We have convincing evidence that, just as previous generations always believed; a good tan is quite healthy for a number of reasons.

There are other problems with sunscreens, too. They block nearly all production of the only vitamin that is also an essential hormone, vitamin D. They dramatically worsen the epidemics of vitamin D deficient diseases of the modern era. Many of these commercial preparations have hormone-mimics that can wreck havoc on your delicate endocrine system. And, worst of all many chemicals used to block UV radiation are themselves carcinogenic!

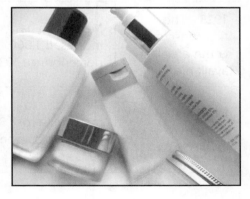

When you take a closer look at sunscreens, you'll see that their regular use will damage your health more than they will protect your skin. And, you'll find natural alternative strategies to avoid both these chemicals and getting sunburned.

Skin Cancer Skyrockets as Sunscreen Use Increases

The first sun-related skin lotions were introduced as early as 1928 as tanning lotion. The goal was to block the rays that burn you so you could stay in the sun without burning. A few years later, the melanoma rate began to rise. Many more tanning lotions hit the market in the early 1960s and a few years after that the melanoma rate zoomed. Rising melanoma rates became hot news.

Seeing a commercial opportunity, the makers of tanning lotions repositioned their products as "sunscreen." They began funding the Sun Police with their anti-sun dogma. Since then, melanoma cases have continued to rise and sunscreen sales continue to climb.

Chemical Sunscreen and Skin Cancer		
Milestone	**Impact**	**Link with Vitamin D**
1928 – The first sunscreen commercially available	Melanoma has increased 1,800 percent since 1930	Direct result of severe vitamin D deficiency.
Early 1970's – Sunscreen more widely used	Death due to melanoma rose 34 percent between 1973 and 1992	Severe vitamin D deficiency causes calcium to be pulled from the bones.

Throw Away Cancer-Causing Sunscreens

Last 30 years – sunscreen use has increased dramatically	Rates of skin cancer skyrocketed	Adequate vitamin D helps prevent the condition.
Sunscreen is now a multi-billion dollar industry	Skin cancer is now the most common cancer in the United States	Vitamin D builds both bone strength and balance reducing falls.

Despite widespread dependence on sunscreen, cases of malignant melanoma continue to climb.[1] Some evidence suggests that the sunscreen themselves increase the risk for melanoma.[2] Countries where sunscreen receives the heaviest promotion also have the fastest rising rates of melanoma.[3]

What Are Sunscreens Doing to Your Skin?

To understand how sunscreen affects your skin cancer risk, you'll need to understand a bit about the how these sunscreens prevent sunlight from burning your skin.

You may remember from high school science that all the colors of the rainbow make up the visible light spectrum but that there are other light frequencies that you can't see. Ultraviolet (UV) light falls just beyond the visible spectrum. We can divide this UV light into 3 groups based on their wavelengths:

1. **UVA (Near UV).** These rays make up 90 to 95 percent of the sunlight that reaches the earth. They have a long wavelength. They penetrate your skin deeply and are primarily responsible for the tanning response in your skin. The atmosphere has a minimal affect on UVA light, so your skin gets exposed

to this kind of light throughout the day. Overexposure to UVA can cause cellular damage.

2. **UVB (Mid UV).** These rays make up 5 to 10% of the sunlight reaching the earth. UVB rays have a shorter wavelength than UVA rays. They trigger vitamin D synthesis in your skin and are responsible for sunburns. The amount of UVB light that reaches your skin depends on the angle of the sun's rays. Therefore, at higher latitudes UV-B can only penetrate your skin during the midday hours.

3. **UVC (Far UV).** These are the shortest wavelengths and would rapidly burn your skin if they penetrated the atmosphere. However, the atmosphere very effectively filters out UVC light. UVC is a potent germicide and kills viruses and bacteria in the atmosphere.

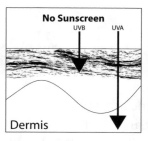 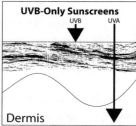 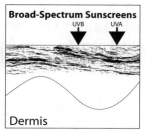

Sunscreens work in one of two ways. They either absorb these UV light rays or deflect them. Commercial sunscreen products use chemicals to do this. You may find many different chemicals in commercial sunscreen lotions but they all use a relatively few number of compounds to actually absorb or deflect UV light.

Throw Away Cancer-Causing Sunscreens

Inconvenient Truth Ignored

Epidemiologist Marianne Berwick, of the Memorial Sloan-Kettering Cancer Center in New York, thoroughly reviewed the ten best to-date studies on sunscreens and cancer incidence. Her results? ***"There is no evidence that use of sunscreen at any age offers any real protection against malignant melanoma"***, the most dangerous form of skin cancer.

She reported her results at the 1998 annual meeting of the American Association for the Advancement of Science. Yet, dermatologists and other Sun Police immediately went on a public offensive encouraging everyone to continue to wear sunscreen, warning that skin cancer would soar if people stopped wearing it.

Most sunscreens use one or more modifications of the following basic chemicals: octinoxate, oxybenzone, octisalate, and titanium dioxide.

Sunscreen and the Epidemic of Skin Cancer

Sunscreens may be part of the cause of our recent epidemic of skin cancer. There are a number of very compelling reasons to implicate sunscreens:

1. Sunscreens effectively stop your skin from protecting itself with melanin.

2. Sunscreens block nearly all your production of cancer-protecting vitamin D.

3. Many chemicals in sunscreen are proven carcinogens (cancer-causing agents).

4. Estrogen mimics in sunscreens cause hormonal disruption and promote tumor growth.

5. Sunscreens don't block all the different frequencies of sunlight sometimes making exposure to cancer causing UV frequencies worse.

1) Sunscreens block your body's production of protective melanin – There is no scientific evidence whatsoever that tanning is a direct risk factor for any disease. There is evidence, however, that a tan is healthy.

One particular study showed that increasing content of melanin in the skin is inversely correlated with the amount of DNA damage that occurs when that skin is exposed to excessive UV radiation.[4] In other words, the tan produced by sunlight protects you from damage from that sunlight.

2) Sunscreen blocks your production of vitamin D – Sunscreens prevent the production of your body's most potent anti-cancer defense, vitamin D. A sunscreen with an SPF of 8 reduces your ability to produce vitamin D by more than 95 percent. A sunscreen with an SPF of 15 reduces vitamin D production by more than 99 percent.[5]

Sunscreen also inhibits your body's natural tanning response. The melanin produced when sunlight strikes your skin protects against sun damage. If you use sunscreen regularly, you are more likely to burn without it.

3) The chemicals in sunscreen are carcinogenic – Chemical sunscreen contains unnatural fats, oils and chemicals. When you apply these to your skin, they can cause free radicals to form.

Cancer-causing Chemicals in Commercial Sunscreens	
Chemical	**Effects**
PABA (also known as octyl-dimethy and padimate-O)	When exposed to sunlight, it attacks DNA and causes genetic mutation.
Octyl-methoxycinnamate (OMC)	Toxic to and can kill cells.
Octyl-dimethyl-PABA (OD-PABA) Benzophenone-3 (Bp-3) Homosalate (HMS) Octyl-methoxycinnamate (OMC) 4-methyl-benzylidene camphor (4-MBC).	Mimic estrogens, causing disruption of real hormone and stimulate cancer cells to grow.

If you look at the label of your sunscreen, you will probably find a chemical known as PABA or padimate-O or one of its close relatives. It is one of the most common ingredients in commercial sunscreens. PABA produces genetic mutations that can lead to cancer, the very thing that sunscreen sellers claim to protect you from with these products.

Even more incredibly, PABA is mostly inert until it becomes illuminated. Exposure to sunlight *causes it to become carcinogenic*. After exposure to UV radiation in sunlight, PABA or padimate-O attacks and damages DNA.[6, 7]

Sunscreens Actually Take Away Your Natural Protection!

What sunscreen makers don't tell you is that sunscreen can rob you of your very best protection against skin cancer – vitamin D and melanin.

- A sunscreen with SPF 15 reduces your vitamin D production by more than 99%!
- Sunscreens inhibit production of your body's natural sun protector melanin.

In addition, many sunscreens protect you only from UV-B rays. These are the rays that cause sunburn. However, it is the UVA rays, which penetrate deep into the skin, which are associated with skin cancer. Without sunscreen, you would generally not be able to stay in the sun long enough for these rays to do damage. But by short circuiting your body's natural "red alert" sunscreen wearers often stay in the sun for hours and hours, all the while, fully exposed to UVA radiation.

According to a study published in the journal *Mutation Research*, "Any padimate-O in contact with the cells substantially increases indirect damage (to DNA)… We estimate that applying an SPF-15 sunscreen which contains padimate-O to human skin followed by exposure to only 5 minimum erythemal doses (MED) of sunlight could… increase strand breaks (DNA) in cells under the epidermis by at least 75-fold compared to exposure to 1 MED in the absence of sunscreen."[8]

An article in the St. Louis Post Dispatch reported that 14 out of 17 sunscreens containing PABA could be carcinogenic when used in the sun.[9] And a study in Great Britain looked at the tendency of PABA (padimate-O) to induce genetic mutation. The researchers stated:

"Chemically speaking, it is identical to an industrial chemical that generates free radicals when illuminated. It is harmless in the dark but mutagenic in sunlight, attacking DNA directly... As mutagens may be carcinogenic, our results suggest that some sunscreens could, while preventing sunburn, contribute to sunlight-related cancers." [10]

Another study found that while most chemicals in sunscreens protect against sunburn, they don't protect against other damage caused by radiation.[11] Because sunscreen makes it seem fine to spend extensive time in the sun, it can encourage you to overdo your sun exposure.

4) Estrogen mimics in sunscreen promote tumor growth – You may not realize that many of the chemicals used in the sunscreen industry mimic the effects of hormones in the body.

Xenoestrogens (foreign estrogens) are among the most common of these chemical hormones. Estrogen-mimicking chemicals stimulate tumor growth and promote the spread of cancer cells. But that's not all. These gender benders can also cause a decline in male sperm

Gender-Bending Chemicals?

Recently, a team of Swiss researchers have found gender-bending chemicals that mimic the effect of estrogen are common in sunscreens which trigger developmental abnormalities in rats. One of the most common sunscreen chemicals, 4-MBC, had a particularly strong effect. When the research team mixed olive oil and applied it to rat skin, it doubled the rate of uterine growth well before puberty.

Researchers worry that the large amounts of sunscreen used by bathers, especially children, could dramatically increase this exposure. They also state the other 25 chemicals used in sunscreens should also be tested for hormonal activity. For the moment, they do not advise people to ditch sunscreens completely, but suggests that sunblocks like zinc oxide might make a healthier alternative.

count, trigger early puberty in girls, and induce feminine characteristics in men.

A Swiss study published in 2001 in *Environmental Health Perspectives* found five chemicals commonly in sunscreens that behave like estrogen.[14] These five xenoestrogens are:

1. Octyl-dimethyl-PABA (OD-PABA)
2. Benzophenone-3 (Bp-3)
3. Homosalate (HMS)
4. Octyl-methoxycinnamate (OMC)
5. 4-methyl-benzylidene camphor (4-MBC)

In laboratory testing, all of these chemicals behaved like strong estrogens, causing cancer cells to grow more rapidly. We also know that when these chemicals are combined they can have a synergistic effect. In other words, two "weak" xenoestrogens can produce a very strong response. Look at ingredients and avoid these in your next bottle of sunscreen.

Safer Alternative Sunscreen?

Some sunscreen producers tout titanium dioxide as a safe physical sunscreen because it reflects and scatters UV radiation. You should choose this above chemicals that are more toxic but even it might not be completely safe. A number of studies show that when illuminated by sunlight TiO_2 causes free radical formation[12] and can initiate DNA damage both in vitro and in human cells.[13]

Probably your safest option is to choose a sunscreen that contains zinc oxide. This is a physical, rather than chemical, sunblock and we know of no studies which show it to cause cell damage.

5) Sunscreen does not block all the rays of the sun – Most sunscreens block only the UVB rays that burn your skin. They allow you to stay in the sun for hours without burning, while your skin soaks up the highly penetrating UVA radiation. Some sunscreen manufacturers now make "broad spectrum" sunscreens that protect against both UVA and UVB rays. But for many years they were not available at all, while these "experts" encouraged increased and imbalanced and possibly deadly UVA exposure.

Studies show that sunscreen users spend more time in the sun because sunscreens short circuit your skin's natural alarm system – the irritation and pain accompanying sunburn. And sunscreens give a false sense of security that promotes overexposure – especially to UVA rays.

Unfortunately, most people believe that sunburn protection equals skin cancer protection. Actual evidence suggests to the contrary - that excessive exposure to non-burning UVA rays not blocked by common sunscreens induces skin cancers including the deadly melanoma variety.[16]

Should You Be Concerned about Chemicals in Your Sunscreen?

Clinical studies show that chemicals in sunscreen significantly penetrate the skin and enter the bloodstream. This means that these chemicals exert their toxic influences not only on the skin, but throughout the body. Especially when you follow the seller's advice to apply generous amounts every hour or two.[15] Put it this way... if you wouldn't drink it, why would you put it on your skin? The effect is just about the same.

Sunscreen: Snake Oil of the 21st Century?

For decades, sunscreen manufacturers have been labeling and advertising their products as protection against skin cancer. As you now know, not only do these products not protect against skin cancer, there is very good evidence that they *cause* it.

This is the motivation behind a new class action lawsuit filed in California against many of the popular sunscreen brands like Coppertone, Hawaiian Tropic, Banana Boat, Bull Frog and Neutrogena.

The lawsuit questions the effectiveness of sunscreens and the honesty of the sunscreen manufacturers' marketing. In their complaint, the plaintiffs call sunscreen the "snake oil of the 21st century." And from what we've seen, this appears to be the case.

Don't be Fooled by Promotional Hype

Even if your sunscreen boasts that it is now "broad spectrum," chemical UVA sunscreens only have a sun protection factor (SPF) of about 4. One study concluded that 90% of melanoma is caused by UVA light.[17] Don't count on sunscreens to protect you from UVA rays.

Sunscreen May Contribute to Cancer – Sensible Sun Exposure Fights Cancer

Sunscreens are not the hero you've been led to believe. Sunscreens abort many of the natural processes that your body uses to protect you and keep you well. In addition, many of the chemicals in commercial sunscreens are carcinogens – linked to cancer in research.

Whenever possible, choose not to use sunscreen. Instead use the common sense we used for eons. Get out of the sun before you start to burn. Cover up with protective clothing and seek shade when necessary. In the next chapter we'll summarize all of the safe sun practices that can help you make good decisions about the sun.

Try These Natural Sunscreens

There are several natural alternatives to sunscreen. You can actually find numerous options online. The important thing is that you test them gradually to make sure that they work with your skin type and to measure their effectiveness so you know how often to reapply.

Lotions containing vitamin C and vitamin E will protect your skin from UV related cellular damage, so they present one option.[18] There has not been research done on how well these prevent sunburn though, so use caution.

Sunscreens with zinc oxide as the active ingredient go on thick, but they are safe and effective. Zinc oxide protects against both UV-A and UV-B rays, and zinc oxide remains stable even when exposed to UV radaition unlike the active ingredients found in most sunscreens.[19]

Protect Yourself Without Sunscreen

Depending on your skin type, you won't need sunscreen if you're going to be in the sun for a shorter period than it takes your skin to burn.

If you're going to spend more time outside, here are a few more ways you can protect yourself from sunburn:

- Use a sun umbrella or sit in the shade.

- Wear a broad-brimmed hat, long-sleeved shirt, and long pants to decrease sun exposure. Tightly woven clothing provides the best protection.
- Take a break by going inside. Visit a local shop, go enjoy a coffee, or check out a local gallery.

If you're going on a daylong snorkeling trip or other adventure that involves long-term sun exposure, look for the most natural, chemical-free sunscreen that you can find. Test the sunscreen *before* you'll be in the sun all day to make sure it works for your skin type. Pay close attention to how often you need to reapply – especially if you're going to be in the water. Check often to make sure you are not burning.

Protect Your Skin with Grape Seed Extract

Researchers from the University of Alabama told attendees at the 233rd national meeting of the American Chemical Society that hairless mice supplemented with proanthocyanidins extracted from grape seed had 65 percent fewer skin tumors than mice not supplemented with the compounds.

The research adds to a small but expanding number of other studies that suggest the grape seed extracts may benefit skin "from within".

According to the European School of Oncology, there are approximately 460,000 new cases of skin cancer in Europe each year, with survival rates improving thanks to more awareness and earlier detection.

If you're going to be outside for a little longer than usual, use a natural sunscreen on your most sensitive areas, usually the face, shoulders, backs of the legs, and tops of the feet. You don't always need to slather sunscreen everywhere. Give some thought to how much exposure you're going to get, and act accordingly.

Throw Away Cancer-Causing Sunscreens

(Endnotes)

1 Bastuji-Garin, S, Diepgen, TL. (2002). <u>Cutaneous malignant melanoma, sun exposure, and sunscreen use: epidemiological evidence.</u> *Br J Dermatol.* 146 Suppl 61:24-30.

2 Annals of Epidemiology, Jan 1993

3 Garland, CF, et al. (1992). <u>Could sunscreens increase melanoma risk?</u> *American Journal of Public Health.* 82(4):614.

4 Tadokoro, T, et al. (2003). <u>UV-induced DNA damage and melanin content in human skin differing in racial/ethnic origin.</u> *FASEB J.* 17(9):1177-9. Epub 2003 Apr 8.

5 Holick, MF. (2004). <u>Vitamin D: importance in the prevention of cancers, type 1 diabetes, heart disease, and osteoporosis.</u> *Am J Clin Nutr.* 79(3):362-71.

6 Hodges, ND, et al. (1976). <u>Evidence for increased genetic damage due to the presence of a sunscreen agent.</u> *J Pharm Pharmacol.* 28:53.

7 McHugh, PJ, Knowland, J. (1997). <u>Characterization of DNA damage inflicted by free radicals from a mutagenic sunscreen ingredient and its location using an in vitro genetic reversion assay.</u> *Photochem Photobiol.* 66:276.

8 Gulston, M, Knowland, J. (1999). <u>Illumination of human keratinocytes in the presence of the sunscreen ingredient Padimate-O and through an SPF-15 sunscreen reduces direct photodamage to DNA but increases strand breaks.</u> *Mutat Res.* 444(1):49-60.

9 Allen, W. (1989). Suspected carcinogen found in 14 of 17 sunscreens. *St Louis Post Dispatch.*

10 Knowland, J, et al. (1993). <u>Sunlight-induced mutagenicity of a common sunscreen ingredient.</u> *FEBS Lett.* 324:309.

11 Wolf P, et al. "Effect of sunscreens on UV radiation-induced enhancement of melanoma growth in mice," *J Natl Cancer Inst* 1994; 86(2): 99-105

12 Warner, WG, et al. (1997). <u>Oxidative damage to nucleic acids photosensi-tized by titanium dioxide</u>. *Free Radic Biol Med*. 23:851.

13 Dunford R, et al. (1997). <u>Chemical oxidation and DNA damage catalysed by inorganic sunscreen ingredients.</u> *FEBS Lett*. 418:87.

14 Schlumpf , M, et al. (2001). <u>In vitro and in vivo estrogenicity of UV screens.</u> *Environmental Health Perspectives*. 109(3):239-44.

15 Sarveiya V, et al. "Liquid chromatographic assay for common sunscreen agents: application to in vivo assessment of skin penetration and systemic absorption in human volunteers," *J Chromatogr B Analyt Technol Biomed Life Sci* 2004; 803(2): 225-31

16 Moan, J, et al. (1999). <u>Epidemiological support for an hypothesis for melanoma induction indicating a role for UVA radiation.</u> *Photochem Photobiol*. 70:243.

17 Setlow, RB. (1999). <u>Spectral regions contributing to melanoma: a personal view.</u> *J Investig Dermatol Symp Proc*. 4:46.

18 Eberlain-Konig B, Ring J. (2005) Relevance of vitamin C and E in cutaneous photoprotection. *J Cosmet Dermatol,* 4(10): 4-9

19 Kullavanijaya P. (2005) Photoprotection *J Am Acad Dermatol*; 52

CHAPTER SIXTEEN

Enjoy Safe Sun Now

*"I am convinced beyond any shadow of a doubt that
as long as you avoid being sunburned, sun exposure
at noon on uncovered skin, is one of the healthiest
things you can do for your body."*

– Dr. Joseph Mercola

As you have now seen, sunlight is not something to be feared and shunned but rather a life-giving force that should be enjoyed, celebrated and respected. Sunshine brings you a host of life-protecting properties, helping you avoid some of the most tragic diseases of our modern-day world.

That doesn't mean you should throw common sense out the window. Staying in the sun too long without protection can cause blistering sunburns that damage your skin. The key is moderation. The amount of sun you need to produce vitamin D can be obtained in as little as ten to fifteen minutes a day, depending on where you live, your skin type, the time of year and your climate.

Get Enough Vitamin D Year Round

Sun is the best source of vitamin D, but for most of us in the US, it's impossible to produce enough from the sun throughout the year. Only UVB rays convert cholesterol in the skin to vitamin D, but most UVB rays are filtered by the atmosphere in high latitudes.

How much UVB light you receive is based on a combination of factors including the time of day, time of year and latitude.

1. **Time of day** – The most UVB rays are present when the sun is highest at noon.

2. **Time of year** – In northern latitudes, it is virtually impossible to get enough vitamin D from sunlight during the winter months. Those in the northern latitudes would benefit from supplementation. During the summer, the best hours to maximize vitamin D are during the times of the day the Sun Police say to avoid – from 10 am to 2 pm.

3. **Altitude** – Ultraviolet intensity increases 4 percent to 5 percent for every 1,000 feet in altitude you ascend. You'll get a sunburn faster in the mountains than at sea level.

4. **Industry** – Pollution, smog and ozone can block UVB.

5. **Climate** – People who live in cloudy climates with long winters are almost surely not getting enough vitamin D.

You Don't Need to Burn to Get Your Vitamin D

How long does it take for your skin to turn pink? If a large part of your body is exposed, you'll only need about 25% of that time to produce the equivalent of taking 20,000 units of vitamin D by mouth.

If your skin doesn't burn, it doesn't mean you need extra time in the sun. One very useful way to figure out the amount of sunshine you need to get adequate levels of vitamin D is to have your blood vitamin D level tested by a physician.

Enjoy Safe Sun Now

How Can I Get Enough Sun to Produce Vitamin D?

Provided that you are at a latitude where and time of year when UVB rays are present, with a little common sense, you can get enough sun to produce vitamin D without damaging your skin. Here are a few guidelines that researchers have recommended:

- One study found that people need 20-120 minutes a day, depending on your skin type and color. If you are fair, you'll want to spend less time in the sun. Darker skinned people need more time to produce vitamin D.

- In warm weather, about 10-15 minutes of direct sun two to three times a week can produce sufficient vitamin D for fair-skinned people. If you have a good tan or a darker complexion, you'll need more sun... up to two hours worth.

- In order to achieve optimal levels of vitamin D, 85 percent of body surface needs exposure to prime midday sun.

Five Steps to Safe Sunbathing

Here are five steps to get sun safely, improve your health and reduce your risk of skin cancer:

1. **A little sun goes a long way** – At the right time of day and year, it takes very little time in the sun to maximize the benefits to your health. Well before your skin even turns pink, your vitamin D production is maximized. Staying in the sun longer than this will not increase your levels of vitamin D.

2. **Obey the laws of good nutrition** – Watch your diet and eat whole foods, not refined, and plenty of fruit and vegetables. The anti-oxidants and nutrients in a fresh, well-rounded diet will help protect your skin from any superficial damage.

3. **Don't ever burn** – You should get sun gradually and consistently over a long period of time. If you are sensitive to sun, you may start out by only exposing small parts of your body, building up to more exposure. Never allow your skin to burn.

   Most people get sunburned because they are so eager for a tan they overdo it. Don't ever bake in the heat, and never spend too long in the sun at one time. Frequent short exposures produce much better results for your health than prolonged exposure. If practical, you should spend a few minutes in the sun several times each day.

4. **Know your skin type** – Those who have very fair skin and burn easily have a higher risk of skin cancer. But even for these people, it is safe to be in the sun… just use your common sense. Sensitivity is the deciding factor. Also, remember that children have more sensitive skin than adults.

5. **Look for alternatives to sunscreen** – Sunscreen prevents the formation of vitamin D, it is toxic and it keeps you in the sun longer than you should be.

Skin Type	Sun History	Example
I	Always burns easily, never tans, extremely sun sensitive skin	Red-headed, freckles, Irish/Scots/Welsh
II	Always burns easily, tans minimally, very sun sensitive skin	Fair-skinned, fair-haired, blue-eyed Caucasians

III	Sometimes burns, tans gradually to light brown, sun sensitive skin	Average skin
IV	Burns minimally, always tans to moderate brown, minimally sun sensitive	Mediterranean-type Caucasians
V	Rarely burns, tans well, sun insensitive skin	Middle Eastern, some Hispanics, some African-Americans
VI	Never burns, deeply pigmented, sun insensitive skin	African-American

How Can I Protect Myself if I Don't Use Sunscreen?

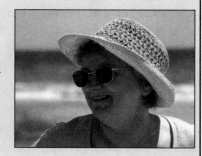

- Use an umbrella, or go inside, or seek shade.
- Wear a broad-brimmed hat, long-sleeved shirt, long pants, and sunglasses to decrease sun exposure.
- Tightly woven clothing provides the best protection. Shield yourself with clothes.
- Use an umbrella or wide brimmed hat at the beach.

Going on a daylong snorkeling trip and not sure how to protect yourself? Look for the most natural, chemical-free sunscreen that you can find. Test the sunscreen *before* you'll be in the sun all day to make sure it works for your skin type. Check often to make sure you are not burning.

What to Do When You Get Sunburned?

In the event that you do get a sunburn, you can take immediate action to prevent damage to your skin.

First, choose one of the topical lotions recommended in chapter 7 and slather it on generously. It's best to choose a water rather than oil-based lotion for this as oils can trap in the heat of the sunburn. Water-based lotions will allow you skin to breathe better.

Next, take an extra gram of vitamin C before going to bed and 400 IU of vitamin E. The anti-inflammatory property of vitamin C can help your sunscreen to heal better and the antioxidant power of both vitamins will help prevent cellular damage.

Enjoy the Sun Safely

Your body has been uniquely engineered to live in the sun. Sunshine reacts with the cholesterol in your skin to start the process of creating activated vitamin D, a hormone that works in the body in an assortment of health-building and disease-preventing ways.

Sunshine also helps your body make melanin, which protects the skin from damage. To let us know when we've spent too much time in the sun, our body begins to turn pink – warning us that it's time to get out of the sun and seek shelter.

You should have an enjoyable, balanced relationship with the sun. Remember sunlight:

- Boosts your vitamin D levels cutting your risks for more than 17 kinds of cancer.

- Lowers your cholesterol and blood pressure.

- Regulates your blood sugar reducing your risk of diabetes.

- Enhances your sexual desires and performance.

- Balances your hormones.

- Lifts your mood.

- Supports your immune system.

- Builds strong bones.

Sunlight can even enhance your ability to learn. There is nothing more natural than time spent in the sun.

The sun police would have you hide from your native sun. They try to scare you with deceitful campaigns based on slivers of half-truths. While their real motive is to sell more sunscreens.

Don't you believe them!

Enjoying the sun is not only every man, woman and child's birthright, it's natures gift to you for a longer, happier and healthier life.

So get out your front door. Soak up some free health rays.

CHAPTER SEVENTEEN

Questions on Sunlight and Health Answered

Don't doctors and researchers have a good reason telling us to avoid sun exposure?

> While it's true that doctors and researchers have good intentions when they recommend you avoid the sun, research results do not support this position. The studies that suggest that ultraviolet is dangerous to your skin and eyes didn't use circumstances that support the position that all sun exposure is dangerous. Review studies looking at lifestyle habits and cancer risks find that people who work and play outdoors have lower incidence of cancer including skin cancer.

Has the sun always been regarded a health hazard?

> For decades doctors recommended sunbathing to patients with rickets, tuberculosis, hypertension, rheumatoid arthritis, and cancer. Some doctors built facilities in the mountains designed specifically around sun therapy.

Why does this book say staying indoors is unnatural and unhealthy?

> If you look at the history of humankind, we have lived outside for most of it. Think of our evolution since we moved from the equator like a single day. On that scale, we've only covered ourselves in clothing within the last several hours. We only began working indoors in the last few minutes. And just seconds ago, sunscreen became

popular. From an evolutionary perspective, people are designed to be out in the sun.

Why is sunlight so important?

There are many reasons. One of the most important reasons sunlight is important is that it triggers the synthesis of vitamin D in your body. Vitamin D is a powerhouse hormone/vitamin combination. Every system in your body needs it for a number of vitally important functions. Since we've begun avoiding the sun, vitamin D deficiency is common and on the rise.

How much sun should I get?

Like most things in life, moderation is key when it comes to sun exposure. You should try to go out in the sun without sunscreen and with a lot of your skin exposed at least three times each week. You should spend 20 minutes to two hours in the sun each time depending on your skin type. Fairer skinned people need less sun than darker skinned people. One rule to never break: Don't ever stay out long enough to burn.

If the sun is so good for you, why do so many dermatologists recommend you avoid it?

Many dermatologists believe they are giving out good advice because skin cancer rates are on the rise. However, there is simply more to good health and sun exposure than skin cancer. And there is more to skin cancer than just sun exposure. The bottom line is that there is a profit motive driving the sun avoidance trend. Sunscreen is a big business, and major sunscreen producers make big donations to professional dermatology organizations.

How does the sun make vitamin D?

When sunlight strikes your skin, it changes pre-cholesterol molecules into cholecalciferol, or vitamin D3. Your body uses this vitamin D3 to make activated vitamin D, which every cell in your body uses to fight disease and maintain your good health.

What are some of the ways my body uses vitamin D?

Vitamin D helps regulate calcium levels in the blood, which helps keep your bones and teeth strong. It's crucial for cells to reproduce properly. It's part of your body's system of energy metabolism. It's important to healthy muscles – your heart is a muscle and vitamin D helps it keep a healthy rhythm. It helps to balance your hormones. The list goes on.

How do I know if I have a vitamin D deficiency?

You should have a blood test done for 25-hydroxyvitamin D. If your levels are below 45 nanograms per milliliter of blood (ng/mL), then they are below optimum. Vitamin D deficiency is officially classified as anything under 20 ng/mL.

What are the risk factors for a vitamin D deficiency?

There are several: location, age, skin type, weight, and lifestyle. If you live anywhere north of Atlanta, Georgia, you are at risk of becoming vitamin D deficient in the winter months. The older you get the harder it is for your body to make vitamin D, so you need more sunlight. Darker-skinned people need more sun to make adequate amounts of vitamin D. Overweight people don't make as much vitamin D. People who work indoors and stay indoors or who only go out after applying sunscreen are usually deficient.

Can I take a vitamin D supplement?

Yes. Sunlight is the best source of vitamin D, but you can take a supplement. In the wintertime, if you live far from the equator, you should take a supplement. Choose only supplements that use vitamin D3 rather than synthetic vitamin D2. The most natural source of supplemental vitamin D is cod liver oil. One tablespoon of cod liver oil each day is enough to keep your vitamin D levels in the optimum range.

Is it possible to take too much vitamin D?

Yes, but it's hard to do. The government recommended daily intake is set far lower than what your body needs. If you use a natural supplement and take between 1500 and 2000 IU each day, then you will be fine. Avoid vitamin D2 supplements as they can become toxic more quickly. It is not possible to get too much vitamin D from the sun.

Doesn't the sun cause skin cancer?

While it's true that repeated sunburns contribute to basal cell and squamous cell skin cancers, the evidence linking sun exposure to dangerous melanoma is less clear. Basal cell and squamous cell cancers are both superficial – they are easily treated and fatal only in the rarest of circumstances. Melanoma is a deadly form of skin cancer that spreads easily to other parts of the body. Much of the evidence out there suggests that responsible sun exposure reduces your risk of melanoma.

What are the risks for skin cancer, then?

There are several factors that contribute to skin cancer. They include your history of sunburn, dietary factors, whether or not you smoke, your skin type (fair-skinned people have higher skin cancer risks), and your family history, among other things.

How do I know if I have melanoma?

Melanoma, the most dangerous form of skin cancer, creates a visible lesion on the skin. Often these lesions look like moles. They are usually asymmetrical. They often have a scalloped border rather than a smooth border. They may have color variations. Rather than being a brown mole, they may have red, white, black, brown, blue, and/or tan all in the same lesion. Melanoma lesions are usually larger than moles, and they often evolve either appearing where there was no mole before or going from a flat mole to a raised mole or becoming itchy.

What about premature skin aging?

There is a connection between sun exposure and premature skin aging, but it is much like the connection between sun exposure and skin cancer – just one factor among many. You can keep your skin healthy and young looking by using a skin moisturizer that contains vitamin E, vitamin C, and equol. Also eating a diet rich in antioxidants and monounsaturated fats helps keep your skin youthful and smooth.

What about the sun and other cancers?

Actually the sun dramatically reduces your risk of deadly internal cancers because of the vitamin D it helps your body produce.

Okay, what other diseases does sun exposure help to fight?

Responsible sun exposure helps to reduce risks of heart attack, stroke, and diabetes. It reduces risks of autoimmune diseases like multiple sclerosis and rheumatoid arthritis. Regular sun exposure also helps to fight depression and promotes a healthy level of sexual desire.

It's cloudy a lot where I live... what can I do?

While there is no substitute for the sun, you can make a big difference in your overall health and well being by switching to full spectrum lighting.

I get depressed in the wintertime. What can I do?

Low vitamin D levels and low exposure to natural light cause depression in many people during the wintertime. Make sure you take a natural vitamin D supplement. Also, use full-spectrum lighting in your house and, if possible, where you work. Go outside whenever it is sunny. Also, research shows that an alarm clock that uses light and simulates the dawn can help.

CHAPTER EIGHTEEN

Sun Solution Resource Guide

Micronutrient Information Center –
http://lpi.oregonstate.edu/infocenter/vitamins/vitaminA/

Nonmelanoma Skin Cancer –
http://www.medicinenet.com/skin_cancer/article.htm

Carcinoma (Websters Online) –
http://www.websters-online-dictionary.org/Ca/Carcinoma.html

Vitamin D Council –
http://www.vitamindcouncil.com/

Topix Health Wire (Search on "Vitamin D") –
http://www.topix.net/health/

Medical News Today –
http://www.medicalnewstoday.com/medicalnews.
php?newsid=30769

Discovery Health (Search on "Vitamin D") –
http://health.discovery.com/

General Health Information

Life Extension Foundation – http://www.lef.com/

Dr. Mercola's Site – http://www.mercola.com/

Books

Douglass, W. "Into the Light" Rhino Publishing, 2003

Hobday R. "The Healing Sun: Sunlight and Health in the 21st Century" Findhorn Press, 2000

Hobday, R. "The Healing Sun: Sunlight and Health in the 21st Century" Findhorn Press, 1999

Holick, M. and Jenkins M. "The UV Advantage" ibooks, 2003

Hyde P.J. "Sunlight, Vitamin D and Prostate Cancer" Xlibris Corporation

Hyde, P. "Sunlight, Vitamin D & Prostate Cancer" Xlibris Corporation, 2002

Kime, Z. "Sunlight" World Health Publications,1980

Liberman, J. "Light: Medicine of the Future" Bear & Company, 1991

Lillyquist, M. "Sunlight & Health: The Positive and Negative effects if the Sun on You" Dodd, Mead & Company, 1985

Lorber J. "The Healing Power of Sunlight" Merkur Pub Co

Merrill M. "Vitamin D: Antidote to Winter and the Darkness" Lulu.com

Moritz A. "Heal Yourself with Sunlight" Ener-chi.com, 2007

Ott, J. "Health and Light: The Extraordinary Study That Shows How Light Affects Your Health and Emotional Well-Being" Ariel Press, 1973

Sorenson M. "Solar Power for Optimal Health" Self-published, 2006

Suntips

http://www.newstarget.com/z020353.html

http://www.newstarget.com/008293.html

http://www.medicinenet.com/script/main/art.asp?articlekey=62117

http://www.sciencenews.org/articles/20051217/food.asp

http://www.news-medical.net/?id=15046

http://www.sciencenews.org/articles/20041009/bob8.asp

http://www.newstarget.com/z020785.html

http://www.westonaprice.org/moderndiseases/sunlight-melanoma.html

http://www.newstarget.com/z021606.html

http://www.newstarget.com/z017590.html

http://www.thefreelibrary.com/Are+you+defficient%3f+Too+little
+vitamin+D+puts+more+than+bones+at+risk-a0153358466

http://www.newstarget.com/021016.html

http://www.newstarget.com/021365.html

http://www.newstarget.com/021229.html

http://www.newscientist.com/article/mg17022870.400-out-of-
the-frying-pan.html

http://www.webmd.com/pain-management/news/20031210/lack-
of-vitamin-d-linked-to-pain

http://www.newstarget.com/021583.html

http://nutraingredients-usa.com/news/printNewsBis.asp?id=75279

http://www.worldhealth.net/p/designing-cancer-killers-a-giant-
leap-forward-in-cancer-treatment-2007-02-28.html

Sunscreen Agents

http://www.mayoclinic.com/health/drug-information/DR202782

http://www.emedicine.com/derm/topic510.htm

Sunscreen Alternatives

http://www.smartskincare.com/treatments/topical/lycopene.html

http://www.worldimage.com/blog/archives/000027_sunscreen_dangers.html

http://www.suerussellwrites.com/tomato.html

http://www.laleva.org/eng/2006/08/sunscreen_found_to_generate_harmful_compounds_that_promote_skin_cancer.html

http://www.realself.com/blog/sunscreen.html

http://www.itmonline.org/arts/seabuckthorn.htm

http://www.naturesgift.com/buckthorn.htm

http://www.earthandseaessentials.com/page/page/3383876.htm

http://www.supersalve.com/ingredients-faqs.html

http://www.curls.biz/Pure+Pomegranate+Seed+Oil+Blend++Experience+the+mo-prd-417.html

http://www.kalyx.com/store/proddetail.cfm/ItemID/570153.0/CategoryID/10500.0/SubCatID/725.0/file.htm

Light Contacts

Duro-Test Corporation:
Vita-Lite
http://www.duro-test.com/
1-800-BUY-DURO
(1-800-289-3876)
12401 McNulty Road, Suite # 101
Philadelphia, PA 19154

G.E. Lighting:
Chroma 50
http://www.gelighting.com/na/business_lighting/
education_resources/literature_library/product_brochures/
downloads/attribute/70610_color.pdf
http://www.geappliances.com/?cid=a97
800-GELIGHT
(800-435-4448)
800-626-2000
G.E. Lighting
Product Service
Nela Park
Cleaveland, OH44112

North American Philips:
Colortone 50
http://www.usa.philips.com/
http://www.nam.lighting.philips.com/us/
212-536-0500
Philips United States
Philips Electronics North America Corporation
1251 Avenue of the Americas
New York, NY 10020

Light Contacts

GTE Products Corporation:
GTE-Sylvania
Design 50
http://www.sylvania.com/
800-LIGHTBULB
978-777-1900
North American Headquarters:
100 Endicott Street
Danvers, MA 01923

Ott Light Systems, Inc.:
Ott Light
http://www.betterlite.com/
http://biolightgroup.com/
http://www.biolightgroup.com/SOLhome.html
805-564-3467
800-234-3724
622 W Arrellaga St Apt C
Santa Barbara, CA , 93101-4147

Verilux Corporation:
Complete Line
http://www.verilux.net/
http://www.verilux.net/products/therapy/index.asp
800-786-6850
802-496-3101
Corporate Headquarters
340 Mad River Park, Suite 1
Waitsfield, VT 05673

Light Contacts

Full Spectrum Solutions:
All Products
http://www.fullspectrumsolutions.com/
888-574-7014
Full Spectrum Solutions, Inc.
Customer Service
PO Box 1087
Jackson, MI 49204

Natural Lighting.com:
http://www.naturallighting.com/web/shop.php
888-900-6830
Naturallighting.com
1414 FM 646 RD E
Dickinson, TX 77539

Lumiram:
http://www.lumiram.com/
Lumiram Electric Corporation
615 5th Avenue
Larchmont, NY 10538

Full Spectrum Store:
http://www.fullspectrumstore.com/
888-638-1893
Full Spectrum Store
2151 Twin Creeks Way,
Ronan, MT 59864

Light Contacts

M&M Lighting Company:
http://www.mmlights.com
888-638-1893
M&M Lighting Co.
2151 Twin Creeks Way,
Ronan, MT 59864

Sun-A-Lux:
http://www.sunalite.com
800-339-9572
American Environmental Products
PO Box 11189
6655 Lookout Road, Suite 120
Boulder, CO 80301

True Sun:
http://www.truesun.com/
877-878-3786
True Sun LLC
1803 Hamilton Place
Steubenville, Ohio 43952

The SunBox Company:
http://www.sunbox.com/ContactUs/
800-548-3968
The SunBox Company
19217 Orbit Drive
Gaithersburg, Maryland 20879-4149

Light Contacts

Light Therapy Products:
http://www.lighttherapyproducts.com/products_bulbs.html
651-351-9800
Light Therapy Products
3207 Summer Fields Ct
Stillwater, MN 55082

Colour Energy Corporation:
http://www.colourenergy.com/misc_products.html
604-687-3757
Colour Energy Corporation
2531 Broadway, Suite D1
Everett, WA 98201

Day Light:
Uplift Technologies Inc.
http://www.day-lights.com/fullspectrum.asp
http://www.up-lift.com/contactus/contactus.asp
902-422-0804
19-10 Morris Drive
Dartmouth, NS B3B 1K8
CANADA

References

Vitamin A:

http://www.feinberg.northwestern.edu/nutrition/factsheets/vitamin-a.html

http://waltonfeed.com/self/health/vit-min/a.html

Vitamin C:

USDA National Nutrient Database for Standard References:
http://www.nal.usda.gov/fnic/foodcomp/Data/SR18/nutrlist/
sr18w401.pdf

World's Healthiest Foods:
http://www.whfoods.com/

Vitamin D:

www.whfoods.com

Wild vs. Farm Raised Salmon:

http://newsletter.vitalchoice.com/e_article000760049.
cfm?x=b11,0,w

USDA National Nutrient Data Base:

http://www.nal.usda.gov

http://ibdcrohns.about.com/od/relatedconditions/a/fdavitd_4.
htm

http://health.allrefer.com/alternative-medicine/vitamin-d-8.html

http://ods.od.nih.gov/factsheets/vitamind.asp#h2

http://yourhealth.calgaryhealthregion.ca/Topic.
jsp?GUID=%7B2D84CB6E-4590-45C2-9D9C-FD5F363598A5%7D

http://www.nysopep.org/pdfs/Prevention_VitaminDSources.pdf

Vitamin E:

USDA National Nutrient Database for Standard References:

http://www.nal.usda.gov/fnic/foodcomp/Data/SR18/nutrlist/
sr18w323.pdf

mg to IU conversion formula:

http://www.feinberg.northwestern.edu/nutrition/factsheets/
vitamin-e.html